POST-
TRAUMATIC
GROWTH

POST-TRAUMATIC GROWTH

thriving in the face of adversity

Brenda Ungerland

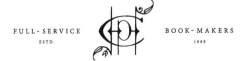

FULL-SERVICE BOOK-MAKERS

ESTD. 1999

COPYRIGHT © 2020
Brenda Ungerland

PUBLISHED BY
Chapel Hill Press, Chapel Hill, NC

....

ISBN 978-1-59715-210-5
Library of Congress Catalog Number 2020906686

First Printing
Printed in the United States of America

Dedicated with love and gratitude
to my beloved
parents, children, and grandchildren
and to all those who strive
to embrace life wholeheartedly
especially our heroic and extraordinary TJ,
triumphant in the face of adversity

CONTENTS

When a water pipe burst in the SoHo loft of an accomplished botanical artist named Margot, most of her paintings, sketches, books, tools, and possessions were completely destroyed. This was particularly traumatic for her since she worked primarily with watercolors. Understandably, the artist was devastated. But something extraordinary happened. After a period of intense grieving, she realized that the experience actually created a sense of spaciousness, an incredible lightness, freedom, and mobility.

Margot went on to conceive a whole new body of work in response to the loss, surpassing what she had previously produced. Her current exhibitions in regional and national museums are a brilliant celebration of her ability to convert personal tragedy into creative expression that both transcends and includes her history.

In the face of unrecoverable losses, her vision has expanded from botanical illustration into unexplored areas of nature art in her ongoing development as a watercolorist. Her commissioned work has vastly increased in the process. The artist might have never recovered from such a traumatic loss. Instead, she evolved.

This is a book about evolving, not as a species but as a person. It's about post-traumatic growth, about thriving, really flourishing throughout one's life, no matter what. It's about coming up against the worst of it—loss, endings, injury, illness, betrayal, anguish, despair, shattering defeat, paralyzing fear—and transforming these excruciating and traumatic realities into experiences of profound growth.

We all share this amazing capacity to emerge from our darkest hour to a better place, more open, loving, whole, freer, and wiser than we were before. It seems extraordinary, and it is. But while change is unstoppable and trauma is unavoidable, transformation remains optional. No guarantees. Only humans can either thwart or catalyze their own human potential and evolutionary development.

Even the grimmest adversity can serve as a pathway to becoming stronger, happier, and more fulfilled. Yet that same adversity can sink you like a stone. Some of us will become immobilized, stuck at an impasse indefinitely, lost in patterns of blame and self-sabotage, distracted with meaningless substitutes, and either stagnate or slowly self-destruct. And tragically, we may never discover what new purpose our life might serve and who we could still become. Statistically, that is the majority of us. But why only some and not others? Why do some of us keep evolving and some of us never change? Conversely, why do some of us remain entrenched in disorders, while others break through and flourish?

The most underexplored, compelling area in human development is, arguably, **post-traumatic *growth***, a phenomenon whose time has come. I should make clear here that, as in all psychological disorders, post-traumatic stress exists on a spectrum from moderate to incapacitating. Severe PTSD must be diagnosed and treated by a licensed mental health professional, for which this book is not, in any way, intended as a substitute.

As a psychologist and seminar leader, I have tracked patterns among individuals in whom moderate trauma preceded profound growth and have witnessed what can and does make a difference, time and time again. From these observations, an empirical model has emerged for turning crisis into expansion, healing, and growth. This model is based directly on commonalities shared by those individuals who actually have succeeded in evolving in the face of adversity. It's a GPS of the soul that has since been applied effectively with countless individuals. While details of our stories are uniquely ours, this practical map offers a way to guide and facilitate the process of inner development, shedding light on how transformational change can happen in one's life.

Each of the seven stages in this blueprint for transformational change has unique challenges, insights, shifts, and turning points: immobilization, unraveling, surrendering, awakening, birthing, integrating, and flourishing. Each stage offers an opportunity to either grow in the process of skillfully managing trauma and change or to become stuck and remain further entrenched. Proceeding to the next level tends to involve mastering certain developmental tasks at each stage and opening to life in previously unconsidered ways. In the process, we continue to become more aware and more adept as we give birth to new dimensions of ourselves. While this capacity for inner expansion often occurs in response to facing intense adversity, it can potentially be experienced throughout our entire lives.

As we all well know, bad things can and do happen to good people. While no one ever sets out to lead a senseless existence—immobilized by fear, diminished by loss, disempowered by defeats, wasting energy on the wrong plan while neglecting the right plan, feeling cramped inside the box—many of us end up doing just that. What is missing when this happens to us? It's not what gets us down but what keeps us down that is at issue here. What is keeping *you* down, despite your best intentions and efforts to bring about change and growth? Many self-help books offer great ideas. But without a realistic blueprint for guidance, we tend to flounder in the dark for way too long, sometimes indefinitely, not really knowing the way forward or out.

Without experience-based input to prepare us for the emotional upheaval that often occurs during each phase, steps to navigate through it, insights to inspire us, and practical skills to persevere, many of us will feel overwhelmed and defeated before we're halfway there. It is precisely when our vulnerability is greatest that we most need a reliable map. This book provides a framework for transformation. It can serve as our **inner**

GPS and private life-coach throughout the process. It provides support and guidance as we forge through high seas of change and loss, consciously evolving, becoming more and more whole.

To the extent that we are consciously working toward becoming more aware and developing our full human potential, we can be regarded as actively participating in our own evolution, co-creating our future, a distinctly human possibility. This is what it means to be whole, fully alive, thriving, and flourishing. In hopes of shedding light on the inner experience of post-traumatic growth and consciously evolving, I have interviewed hundreds of individuals who have successfully recovered from some of the most painful ordeals imaginable: cancer diagnosis, financial ruin, death of a loved one, painful divorce, debilitating injury, life-threatening illness, profound loneliness, recurring addiction, chronic anxiety and depression, and others.

Each of the seemingly ordinary individuals included in this book has emerged through times of unspeakable despair with a sense of triumph and even gratitude for what they learned, how they've grown, and who they became in the process. Against all odds, they have become men and women of remarkable wholeness, love, depth, spirit, and joy. Yet they once thought their life, the life they'd planned and dreamed of, was basically over. And it certainly was. But there was something very different and quite beautiful waiting for them.

As their stories unfold through each phase of their transformative experience, this book offers powerful guiding metaphors for one's own journey. This direct glimpse into the phenomenology of developmental change reveals important insights about how the inner process of profound growth actually occurs. Although each person's challenges are vastly different, a roughly comparable sequence of dynamics and turning points can be seen running through their experience.

In bearing witness, we can only be reassured and inspired by the dramatic changes that can and do take place. It is a messy and often harrowing process. There is within us something dying and something being born. But despite our perceptions to the contrary, we are never totally alone. We do have each other. We are all in this together. We are each other's teachers, "each other's miracle," as poet **Marge Piercy** has said.

Maybe the first step is to realize that we will somehow be held and nourished, often when we least expect it, by a friend or by a perfect stranger—it doesn't matter—or by a moonrise on a river, an evocative poetic metaphor, a stirring cello concerto, stillness in meditation, a great night's sleep, morning sun through our kitchen window, the scent of a ripe plum, by sudden laughter, a field of wildflowers, by one good book that speaks directly to us. Anything can heal us. So first we open to that. We exhale. And then we look for practical inspiration.

Even without a major crisis, many of us will eventually find ourselves asking, "Is this it?" and begin seeking new ways to expand our world. Here the process of self-actualization or personal evolution is actually self-initiated, generated from a place inside us that is tugging at us to grow. It says, "Enough!" Perhaps the life plan that seemed complete has begun to feel narrow and confining. We have a persistent longing to be more alive, more connected, more fulfilled, an impulse to learn, to take on new challenges and experiences. By becoming more informed about the territory of change and more adept at navigating it, we will be honing the skills and developing the traits we need to continue thriving and flourishing throughout our life no matter what.

As a point of clarification, this model of stages and phases has been drawn from two sources: first, from my field research with individuals who have personally succeeded in converting moderate trauma into transformative growth, and second, from the observations of experienced psychologists and psychiatrists who have assisted in this process with private clients. Their professional perspective on the key components involved in profound change sheds further light on both the catalysts and the impediments to post-traumatic growth and transformation.

As with the stages of grieving, loosely defined by **Elisabeth Kubler Ross** in *Death and Dying*, there is naturally lots of overlapping, backtracking, and advancing between phases. This is not a tidy, precise process. However, in my experience working with hundreds of individuals and road-testing this model as a developmental guide, we have found it to be easily as valuable for transcending trauma as the Kubler Ross model has been for grieving, as well as enormously validating and helpful. May it guide and support you on your way.

CHAPTER I

Immobilization—Becoming Stuck

This chapter introduces the first phase, Immobilization, revealing the inevitability of feeling overwhelmed and lost at some point in our life, why this happens to the best of us, and what keeps us stagnating in that dark, painful place far longer than necessary. This is the time to step back from our life and begin the process of honestly acknowledging how it's going.

IN THE BEGINNING

In the beginning, we come into this world exuberant—pure and free, innocent and hopeful, blank as an uncarved block. We spend our early childhood soaking up life, our brains continuously downloading information from our family and cultural environment. We are shaping and reshaping our sense of self in response to everything we experience as children. Even as a tiny infant, we are forming the lens through which we will perceive and interpret the world, drawing conclusions about life, how the world works, who we are, and how we fit into this picture.

In time, some of our experiences will be screened out by this very lens, and others will be amplified. It is through this filtered lens that we will gaze at life, forming our uniquely subjective and personal view of reality. We will carry this filter with us into every challenge, every relationship, every situation, every moment we encounter. Until we recognize this fact, we are operating under the illusion that our take on reality is fully objective, that our viewpoint is entirely logical. Not necessarily. Yet it is on the basis of our inner experiences and subjective impressions that we develop strategies, learn rules, and hold expectations about ourselves and others.

The first half of our adult life is spent basically living out the programming that we have absorbed from our environment, playing out our roles, based on the beliefs and premises of our indoctrination, and still perceiving it all through this somewhat distorted lens. This is the period that Carl Jung describes as the first adulthood, when the primary focus is between one's ego and the world. One of the givens of our early adult life is the perception that responding to what the world seems to be demanding of us means holding up our end of "the contract," which in turn will ensure our happiness. The more we have of XYZ, the better it will be. Knowledge? Status? Wealth? Beauty? Pleasure? Security? Achievement? Control? Whatever we learned was most important.

We make our decisions based on this belief: that our big choices— what we do, where we go, who we marry, how we love, when we play, how we live—are so logical that surely they will make us happy. And they often do, at least for a while. Our choices are based on the firmly held premise that we are doing what we must do to get our life right. And it often seems to be working reasonably well, roughly according to expectation. Until something happens. Suddenly or gradually, something changes, causing us to question everything, radically altering our sense of who and what and where we are.

It can come to us from the outside in the form of an unexpected loss, injury, diagnosis, or discovery, some concrete evidence that shocks us like a lightning bolt into the unknown. And it can just as easily happen more internally in the form of disillusionment, the collapsing of denial, a nagging sense of emptiness, worsening anxiety, self-sabotaging behavior, a sadness that nothing seems to lift. And one day we find ourselves lost, wings broken, adrift in space. Our life feels like a huge mistake, a betrayal of our dreams. "Why me?" we ask. As if this shouldn't be happening. As if this is cruel and unusual punishment. As if it were somehow preventable. "How could this be happening?" we ask, wishing we could explain it to ourselves.

But some crash landings are in store for all of us. It is only a question of when. Why? Because our expectations, inevitably, were based partly on illusions. Some of our most unquestioned premises and givens were destined to unravel to begin with. And when reality fails to meet our deepest expectations, we find ourselves stymied, facing what feels impossible and unsolvable—stuck in the bottom of a deep dark pit, banging our head against the wall.

Although we'd hate to admit it, we feel helpless, frightened, insecure, chaotic, and powerless to change the outcome. Our sense of safety is shattered, at least for the moment. We take this to be a bad thing. And of course, it is very, very painful. But it is also a necessary prelude to meaningful change, drawing us toward our potential for transformational growth. This is precisely the kind of purposeful falling apart that precedes our inner reorganization at a higher level. Disintegration is followed by more advanced reintegration. It is how we all evolve from one level of conscious awareness to the next and the next.

Our illusions are going to break down all on their own in time. Whatever is unsustainable is programmed to eventually collapse. When this happens, we're either going to tighten our grip on "what might have been" (but is not real, not now anyway) and sink with it, resisting reality, becoming and staying depressed about it. Or we're going to enter the mystery. Which means going into the darkness and chaos and trusting the process, trusting that there is a larger story and that this is merely a chapter in it. We may still feel trapped in the bottom of a deep hole, but at least we sense that there is an opening above us and that somehow we will build a ladder to bring us up and out. We may even sense that there is a mysterious kind of intelligence operating in our life, guiding us in ways that are only vaguely perceptible.

Sometimes I go about pitying myself,
and all the time I am being carried
on great winds across the sky.
CHIPPEWA

Does it somehow seem selfish to be following our dream as if it really matters? Usually! Yet in every moment that we spend furthering our own development, we are contributing to the greater good. **Buckminster Fuller** had a word for it. He called this phenomenon "precession," when he described honeybees doing what they do best: gathering nectar for honey, oblivious to the fact that they are making a crucial contribution to nature. Cross-pollination of the entire meadow depends simply on their instinctive comings and goings every day.

What about our instinctive comings and goings, our intuitive callings, when we actually hear them and honor them? What Fuller is suggesting here is that by fulfilling our truest calling, we are by definition serving a higher purpose. Whether we happen to be aware of it is not the point. The bees aren't. It's enough to just be open to it, listening to the still small voice within, and making conscious choices and ongoing adjustments, paying attention to insights and realigning our life in accordance with them.

It takes real courage to open to the reality that is presenting itself, first by acknowledging how different it may be from what we had planned for our life and then by finding ways of opening to new possibilities nonetheless. It is in grieving our losses and relinquishing our unfulfilled dreams that we create essential space for what lies ahead. Composting the broken dreams of our first adulthood is a necessary step in our initiation into what Carl Jung calls the second adulthood.

Here the focus is less on what the outside world seems to be demanding of us and more on the quality of our inner experience, the realm of the self. This shift in perspective lets us off some old hooks and outgrown premises that no longer have meaning. And then it guides us into the sacred ground of what really matters to us, here and now. For all the loss this entails, there is a sense of being liberated from rules that were too confining anyway, keeping us trapped inside a smaller story in shoes that no longer fit.

David Whyte speaks to this at the end of his poem *Sweet Darkness.*

> *You must learn one thing,*
> *The world was made to be free in....*
> *Give up all other worlds except*
> *the one to which you truly belong.*
> *Anything that does not bring you alive*
> *is too small for you.*

Navigating the high seas of transition requires new skills, new tools, and, above all, the passion that can only come from our own vision of how we would love to be, now that so much has changed. Right along with the sadness and fear, loss and chaos, we need to be reconnecting with forgotten parts of ourselves and giving birth to new ones. Now is the time to turn inward for promptings of the soul. "Everything is waiting for you," says poet David Whyte. It has been all along.

> *Deep in their roots all flowers keep the light*
> THEODORE ROETHKE

It can come to us anywhere—in a deep dream or a quiet waking moment, during walks or meditation, on the train or in the shower—anytime there is some free space inside of us. We just need to open a file in our minds and invite it to come to us, to flow into the clearing. And then be patient with the process. The storm may be raging now, but we know the sky will clear again. We can rest our heart on that.

In contrast to the first adulthood when we looked outside ourselves for the answers, we are more and more turning inward now, with an emphasis on the unasked questions instead. This is a time of remembering who we are in our most essential self. We are each endowed with gifts to give and purposes to accomplish that are absolutely unique to our individual self. We are like an acorn endowed with an inner blueprint and everything it needs to become an oak, as **James Hillman** has observed. Often it is not until our shell is broken open through the major and minor devastations of life that we come home to ourselves with new eyes. This too is a seminal part of the journey, part of the experience of self-honoring. "Come home to your soul, never to be led away," says **Hermann Hesse**.

It is from the rubble of what has broken down in our lives that transformation can begin to come forth. Everything in the natural world is engaged in transforming. Seed to plant, plant to rice, rice to human, human to Buddha, it is said. Nothing can or will stay the same. Everything alive is transforming—dying off and blooming, declining and self-regulating, disintegrating and reorganizing, adapting and evolving potentially. Yet only humans, through conscious choice, can reshape their lives in accordance with their vision. The process of emergence begins with a tiny seed, a longing, an impulse, an intuition, an awareness. It feels undeniable and irrepressible. It comes to us in the middle of inevitable crisis, the kind that is waiting for every one of us, although the details will be uniquely ours.

Remember the irrepressible curiosity you felt as a child? The juiciness? Where is it now? In the spirit of trusting the process, please notice that you have taken the action of opening this book. In the pages ahead, you will find yourself engaged in a provocative dialogue with yourself. You will be supported in the actual process of personal transformation, of opening, uncovering, expressing, discovering, taking action, integrating, emerging. And the following **question** is a good place to start:

> *If you woke up today somehow magically*
> *cured of all your inner obstacles,*
> *limitations, hesitations, how would you know?*

- How would you be feeling?
- What would you be doing?
- What would be different about you?

Please consider writing down your responses to these questions, giving yourself permission to dig deeply while recording your initial gut reactions, for your eyes only. It can be extremely helpful to the process of discovering and expressing all that lies in waiting, just below the surface. You are encouraged to spend some time at the end of each chapter making some notes, either here or in your private journal.

ADVERSITY AND PAIN: THE MANY FACES OF CRISIS

Let's begin with some actual case studies to illustrate both the nature of the crisis experienced and the initial reaction of the individuals we will be tracking in the course of this book. While the names and certain details are changed to protect their privacy, the responses of the individuals quoted are largely verbatim. Any resemblance to specific people you may know is purely unintentional and accidental.

CASE STUDIES: DURING THE IMMOBILIZATION PHASE

SARAH Sarah, a 35-year-old sales associate, was leaving a local restaurant one sleeting, icy night in February when an oncoming car lost control and skidded into her, pinning her against a cement wall. Both of her legs were completely smashed to shreds, almost to the hip. The first witness who encountered her vomited instantaneously, an image that would haunt Sarah for years.

She left the hospital's rehab wing several weeks and surgeries later, sitting in a wheel chair, balanced on her thigh stumps. Sarah soon became adept at managing her everyday life at home, building arm strength, and acquiring new skills.

But her emotional healing proved far more elusive. Her inner reality?

"I am horribly mutilated; I am repulsive." Yet, unlike many amputees who live out sheltered and disconnected lives numbed by medications or addictions, Sarah's life opened up in ways she could never have anticipated. She is a stunning inspiration today—joyful, creative, productive, and yes, still chic and slender in her snappy high-tech wheel chair.

How did she move forward from this debilitating trauma, physically and emotionally, against all odds? Moving into and out of each stage of transformation, she came back to life with a passion, amazing herself and everyone who sees her today.

JANE "What amazes me most about staying in a bad relationship is that it was so okay for me for so long. I was always diminishing myself, always thinking it was my fault, thinking I wasn't trying hard enough or just wasn't desirable enough for him. Maybe if I was thinner or smarter or funnier or whatever, then he would be loving toward me." Despite her private anguish, Jane hung in bravely for years on end before facing the need to end her dysfunctional marriage.

She saw it as her life, living with the man she was so committed to, in the only life she had known for 22 years, until she began to realize instinctively that if she didn't get out, she would die. She had spent years in denial, refusing to acknowledge just how much she had given up in order to stay with him and, even worse, how disabled she had become in the process.

In response to his relentless criticism, heartlessness, and mistreatment, she had just kept trying harder. The more Jane did to make the relationship work, the less he seemed to care. The more he disregarded her, the less she came to expect from him. Whenever she raised the question of marriage counseling, he laughed at her. She stopped asking. Years went by. At age 46, she could hardly remember the vibrant, confidant woman she once was.

She had learned to cope with his narcissistic self-absorption and overlook his disrespect, but it was at the grinding expense of her self-esteem and physical well-being. Then one fine day, she woke up and said the unthinkable to herself: "Whatever the cost, emotionally and financially, I am getting out of this." How did she finally bring herself to do what she had needed to do for so long? Her story provides a blueprint for proceeding through the stages.

TED By all outward appearances, Ted, age 44, was a successful civil engineer living his personal dream of the good life: a weekend home, a sailboat, travel, memberships in private clubs. Because of his confident style and increasing net worth, who would guess that just below the surface Ted had a gnawing sense of emptiness and despair?

"How did I get to this place? It can only work if I'm not true to myself; my needs can't matter. It looks like success, but there is no joy in it. It's all work. I can barely remember who I am." Years of overwork, sleep deprivation, anxiety, and self-neglect had begun to compromise his health seriously. Lower back pain, headaches, skin rashes, lack of energy, and digestive problems had plagued him for nearly a decade, despite continuous medical treatment.

Yes, he was a high-performing employee with great intelligence and skills. But he had come to hate his job—the hours, the pressure, and eventually even the work itself. Burned out and depressed, sedating himself on weekends, he saw no feasible alternatives to his lifestyle that seemed acceptable, particularly to his wife. He simply could not afford to switch career paths, financially or emotionally. He felt trapped and stuck, and then he hit the wall. After a major unraveling, he went on to forge a whole new life in synch with his true nature, moving through the stages step by courageous step.

CAROL When her physician scheduled an after-hours meeting with Carol and her husband, she knew instantly that the news would not be good. After endless rounds of lab tests, EKGs, and EEGs, a series of MRIs confirmed the neurologist's diagnosis. Carol, age 36, wife and mother of three young children, did, indeed, have multiple sclerosis.

Her first reaction was panic and devastation. "Oh, my God. My life is ruined. I'll be dependent, pathetic. My husband will leave me, and my children, the poor kids. Why should they be punished? Why should I be punished like this? I can't even think straight."

It was inconceivable to Carol that this would happen to her of all people. "I faked my way in public for five years after the diagnosis, getting worse all the time."

The charade was unsustainable and increasingly detrimental to her mind and her body. Eventually she hit the wall, breaking down, emotionally, physically, and spiritually. What followed, however, was a phase of breaking open and a breaking through that brought her to a place way beyond mere acceptance of her diagnosis and her disabilities.

She went on to embrace the worst and the best of the hand she had been dealt. Carol is now living life wholeheartedly, singing in a church choir with a special stool for when she's unable to stand, cheering at her kids' field hockey games from a wheelchair without hesitation, teaching a nutrition course from her home, and savoring downtime with her husband and close friends. And doing it all with gratitude.

The process was gradual, of course, but once her relationship to her disease began to shift emotionally and cognitively, her declining physical condition began to stabilize along with the severity of her symptoms. She has been able to maintain this remission for more than 10 years now, surpassing all expectations, medically and personally.

BRAD Concerned about preserving his investments in a confusing economic environment, Brad decided to seek the services of a qualified financial adviser. Although accomplished in his field of medicine, Brad, age 54, knew he lacked the depth of knowledge in stock market investments to make informed choices. Hiring an experienced professional to manage his account seemed like the responsible thing to do.

It was his life savings after all, unrecoverable income, and he could not afford to risk losing his hard-earned money on any imprudent financial decisions. After a lengthy search, Brad delegated the management of his portfolio to a financial adviser at a prestigious Wall Street firm with a sense of relief and trust that his assets were now safely invested.

Six months later, when the value of Brad's investments plummeted, the trusted adviser showed her true colors. She had fraudulently exposed his life savings to huge risks in order to garner multiple kickbacks and bonuses for herself. In the end, Brad was left with a small fraction of his original net worth and no real recourse.

"How could this possibly be happening? How could someone so ruthlessly betray my trust and legally get away with it!?" Brad was immobilized with self-recrimination for trusting the wrong person, sadness at the irrevocable loss, and fear for his future life. Despite his initial devastation, Brad began to move diligently through the stages. In the end, he forged a whole new way of living that was quite unlike his past but deeply rewarding in unanticipated ways.

DANIELE Daniele was 17 years old when she was sexually assaulted by an older friend of her extended Latino family, someone she had trusted for years. "After that night, I was lost and confused. Like most rape victims, I felt guilty, as though somehow I was to blame for him having sex with me against my will. I am now aware that any one of us can be violated, no matter our socioeconomic background, race, age, or gender." As the daughter of a physician father and a biochemist mother, Daniele's young life had been blessed with the many intellectual, emotional, cultural, and educational benefits of a good home. Most importantly, she had two very loving parents with solid values who did everything possible to raise a happy and confident young woman.

But her sense of self was utterly shattered by the trauma of rape. It had left her feeling violated, depressed, fearful, disconnected, and withdrawn. He was someone she had known and confided in for years. Daniele's tragedy is all too common. But how her story unfolds amazes and inspires everyone. What she did to transcend the pain and heal her emotional wounds converted her tragic experience into a catalyst for creativity and growth. Today, age 20, she is a public speaker, student leader, activist, and founder of a healing arts initiative.

MIKE Although he'd once been strong and athletic, Mike's years of cocaine abuse had left him gaunt, shaken, and sickly. At only 42, he had already suffered "two mild heart attacks and pneumonia from drug abuse, but I still didn't care if I died. I just wanted those caps. I would stop at the crack house on my way home from work, hang out with my buddies, buying as much as I could. And then we would scatter like rabbits. I was so paranoid about being seen. I would race home and hide in the bathroom, crouched on the floor like an insect. Sometimes I would lace the drugs with vodka until I was launched."

His life was an utter nightmare. Despite his family, his job, and his potential, drugs were all he thought about. But eventually he hit the wall. And then he made his way back, freeing himself from his 20-year enslavement. Today he is an addiction counselor, clear and clean for more than 12 years, leading retreats and workshops. His journey provides compelling evidence that transformation is achievable, phase by phase, even in such extreme circumstances.

JULIE When I first met Julie, an 86-year-old psychiatrist, MD, Ph.D., holocaust survivor, she was trapped in a suicidal depression following the death of her beloved husband. She was ready to end her extraordinary life. She had escaped the Nazi regime first in Vienna in 1938, then in Prague shortly after, and finally in Amsterdam, where she remained hidden in a closet from 1943 to 1945, through the sheltering kindness of a Christian family. Her subsequent post-war years in America with her devoted husband had been the only enduringly positive time in her entire life. His death left her with no reason to go on.

Julie's plan at the time was to end her life as soon as she felt the final impulse. She had everything she needed in place: a self-prescribed prescription, notes, and directives. But she decided to hold off for a month or so and give me the chance to work with her for a few sessions. What followed took place over a period of roughly six years as it turned out, during which Julie explored and moved through all of the phases—from immobilizing depression to a place of openness and, to her amazement, joyfulness.

Slowly proceeding through the wall of silence that she had fiercely maintained for decades, she gave voice to years of repressed outrage, fear, and grief. She made her way back into the darkness of her unwitnessed history, released unexpressed emotion, and gradually emerged with a level of lightness, emotional freedom, and inner peace that she had assumed was completely unattainable.

As Julie revealed her excruciating but triumphant and wildly colorful story in vivid detail for the very first time, she demonstrated, once again, that it's never too late for spiritual healing, never too late to become whole. During those last six years of her life Julie truly evolved. She was able to transcend the anguish of her past, reconnect with the unscathed beauty of her soul, honor her great appetite for life, and even share her outrageous sense of humor with abandon. Bedridden and blind, she nonetheless lived a remarkably full and joyful final chapter, always challenging her intellect and savoring connections with close friends and former patients. She died peacefully, gracefully, totally on her own terms, two weeks after her 92nd birthday. Her final words? "It's all about love."

THE ABYSS

We are both the abyss and the tightrope across the abyss.
FRIEDRICH NIETZSCHE

Let's take a closer look at the bottom. How does being in the abyss of adversity feel to us on the inside? Individual specifics aside, there are certain biological, emotional, and cognitive commonalities involved in how all of us experience crisis or acute stress. What's it like when this is happening? The first phase, immobilization, begins with a negative event or perception that triggers an extreme emotional response. We are stunned, terrified, maybe outraged. We may feel like we're sinking, falling, spinning, crashing, or lashing out with blame. We feel a sense of powerlessness and betrayal. Or we go numb and shut down. Initially, our perception is that we're up against an insurmountable problem, feeling trapped at an impasse, stuck in a no-win nightmare, or hopelessly lost. Our anxiety level is through the roof.

At this point, whether we recognize it or not, we really can't think straight. It's as if fear is obscuring our reasoning powers, which of course it is, temporarily. Here is where we lose our perspective, leaving us blind to important options and possibilities. We experience our life as intensely painful, contracting, narrowing down into a grim spiral from which we fear we may never pull out. We question our past decisions and cringe at the ineffectiveness of our strategies. We may be overcome with resentment and hostility or feel hopelessly derailed and vulnerable.

Regardless of whether we fall into this phase in a sudden trauma or as a last straw, the result is the same: We feel truly overwhelmed. Our confidence is shaken and our optimism is shattered. Our ability to trust in life? Gone. Blocked, anxious, disempowered, and depressed. This is what it's like to become stuck. Here is a generic **composite** of how we're likely to feel and what we tend to say to ourselves, when we are under the influence of elevated anxiety during the immobilization stage:

- I am beside myself ... can't think straight ... how could this happen to me?
- it's unbearable ... impossible ... excruciating ... unfair ... I can't go on
- I'll be devastated if ... I can't believe it ... I can't handle it
- I feel: betrayed ... violated ... humiliated ... broken ... disgraced ... decimated ... useless ... worthless ... abandoned
- Like such a loser ... like a failure ... like I don't matter ... why me?
- Like my life doesn't matter ... like my needs are irrelevant ... it's pointless
- This is killing me ... this situation is out of control ... I am out of control
- What's there to live for? ... What is life about? ... Why is this happening?
- I feel terrified ... obsessed ... depressed ... devastated ... wrecked
- Searching ... grasping ... beside myself ... helpless ... manipulated ... trapped
- I have to get out ... I am confused ... ruined ... irreparably damaged
- This is the worst ... horribly painful ... senseless ... I'm so ashamed
- I don't know who I am anymore ... I wish I were dead ... my life is over
- I have no choice ... life has no meaning now ... there is no point
- I am broken and I can't be fixed

Grim as they are, these are the precise thoughts and words of the very people who went on to triumph, flourish, and amaze themselves. Yet this stage was experienced as a time of such acute crisis that their day-to-day existence felt unbearable.

They may have been exerting tremendous effort in their lives to feel okay, to be happy, motivated to "do the right thing," and bravely deal with their emotional pain; but their sense of crisis at this point was just overwhelming. This is when our previously useful coping mechanisms are either proving insufficient or ineffective, or they may actually be making matters worse. At this point, we have not yet fully grasped either the full magnitude or the true root of the problem.

The immobilization stage can last anywhere from weeks, to months, to years, to an entire lifetime. Certain impediments extend it. They are obstacles to growth, masquerading as helpful. But they only prolong the agony as we attempt to minimize our pain. They are the **reactive behaviors** and unwittingly self-destructive strategies we tend to use when dealing with stress:

- **Patterns of denial, avoidance, and withdrawal:** overworking, hiding out, pretending—all are forms of distracting ourselves from facing what we don't want to look at.
- **Disassociating from what is happening:** going numb, working hard at staying oblivious to the issue that we're not ready to confront.
- **Escape:** self-medicating with alcohol or drugs when too much is still never enough and our behaviors are only exacerbating the problem.
- **Obsessive-compulsive behaviors and thoughts:** This lowers anxiety in the short term at the expense of real progress, and it compromises the quality of our relationships.
- **Mindlessly serving cultural myths that lack meaning:** What made sense at an earlier stage of development may be thwarting or even crippling growth in the present.
- **Various forms of self-betrayal:** These are actions arising from a fear-based mentality that serve only to keep us small, undermining our ability to heal and grow.

Living with elevated levels of anxiety for extended periods of time can lead to fairly predictable side effects, the most common being depression, anxiety disorders, panic attacks, addictive behaviors, stress-related illnesses, etc. These are inevitable manifestations of unhealed emotional pain. The intense distress of remaining stuck in the immobilization phase jeopardizes our well-being, predisposing us to a vast array of stress-related illnesses, from headaches and allergies, to irritable bowel syndrome, digestive disorders, rashes, cardiovascular disease, neuromuscular problems, auto-immune disorders, and chronic pain. The significance of the mind-body connection will be explored more fully at the end of this chapter.

But to sum it up, while the external details of becoming stuck vary widely, our perceptions and emotions tend to have a common thread. In the midst of adversity, we feel immobilized by what seems intolerable and unsolvable as we fluctuate between anxiety and depression. This is the dark night of the soul, described centuries ago:

> *In the middle of the road of my life*
> *I awoke in a dark wood*
> *Where the way was wholly lost*
> DANTE

The following excerpts reveal the voice of despair, tied to *specific situations and individuals*, during their personal experience of the immobilization phase:

"What did I do wrong? What's wrong with me? I felt beaten again, punished, not ready to give up, but I felt devastated. I felt angry, defeated, so depressed."
FRAN, 38-YEAR-OLD WOMAN FACING INFERTILITY

"I suddenly realized I will never recover from this loss. I will never again be able to afford my current way of life. I can't be generous to my kids the way I've been and want to be. I'll probably lose my home. There was an intense feeling of having failed, of searching and feeling lost. It was total confusion inside. I was afraid of not finding a way out, of not surviving this."

BRAD, 54-YEAR-OLD MAN IN SEVERE FINANCIAL CRISIS

"Fear was the operative word. I was scared to death. I was in such emotional pain; the marriage was dead, but it took eight years to go through with it because I was so afraid."

LISA, 47-YEAR-OLD WOMAN DIVORCING AFTER 23 YEARS OF MARRIAGE

"I spent the last 12 years feeling restless and unsatisfied, doing my job, but right on the brink. I was always searching, groping, but going nowhere. My life made no sense. These were not my values. Where did I go wrong?"

TED, 44-YEAR-OLD INVESTMENT ADVISER IN CAREER CRISIS

"Fear. If it hit my trigger point, I was medicating myself again with wine, valium, etc. I was a control freak, always on the edge. I was a know-it-all, tough on the outside, dying on the inside. Everything is deadly serious with me—have fun? What the hell is that?"

DONNA, 42-YEAR-OLD WOMAN IN PERSONAL AND FAMILY CRISIS

"The most depressing part for me was the way people look at you. I was always so terrified of embarrassment, about facing people, always hiding my body. I was so miserable, so alone"

SARAH, 35-YEAR-OLD WOMAN WHO LOST BOTH LEGS IN A CAR ACCIDENT

"I thought something was wrong with me. I was always trying to fix it, always trying to alter myself in some way, for harmony in the marriage, whatever. I tried therapy, tried treating him differently. Nothing helped."

JANE, 39-YEAR-OLD WOMAN IN AN ABUSIVE RELATIONSHIP

"I wanted out every day, fought daily with myself. You reach a level of insanity. My body was craving it; my mind was hating it. I knew this was ruining my life, but I just couldn't stop."

STEVE, 47-YEAR-OLD DENTIST ADDICTED TO PRESCRIPTION DRUGS

"The pain was unbearable. I couldn't stop crying. I knew I was being too needy, but I was out of control. It was beginning to alienate my friends. I felt ashamed and rejected. I felt old, out of shape, and worthless."

MEREDITH, 40-YEAR-OLD WOMAN, RECENTLY DIVORCED

"I felt trapped. My biggest concern was the impact on my children and then the concern that there would be divisiveness and the possibility of a backlash against me. Could this destroy me?"

PAUL, 56-YEAR-OLD MAN ENDING A 30-YEAR MARRIAGE

"To me, initially, this was the major thought: I can't believe this could be happening to me. Most of my values slipped into the backseat: my career, work, socializing."

KIM, 45-YEAR-OLD WOMAN DIAGNOSED WITH BREAST CANCER

"I just couldn't let go. I could never let my guard down. I had to row like hell; I thought that if I ever stopped rowing, I would just go over the edge."

ALISON, 34-YEAR-OLD RECENT WIDOW WITH FIVE CHILDREN

"I started screaming uncontrollably. I was feeling feelings, then not feeling anything, then feeling terrified and all alone."

ANNE, 28-YEAR-OLD WOMAN WHO LOST HER PARTNER IN A CAR ACCIDENT

"I was fully prepared to end my life. I was just waiting for the impulse to commit suicide. My life was torture. My constant thought? Nothing matters now. There is no meaning in my life. I just want to die, not to live another day."

JULIE, 86-YEAR-OLD MD, RECENTLY WIDOWED, IN SUICIDAL DEPRESSION

"I didn't know who I was or anything. I looked in the mirror and wanted to take a knife and cut myself open metaphorically to find out what's inside. That was the intensity of the search."

JONATHAN, 32-YEAR-OLD TEACHER IN AN EXISTENTIAL CRISIS

"I was oblivious, never sober, and with no concept of anything but that way. I knew I was at my bottom, but I really thought I had no way out."

DORIS, 50-YEAR-OLD ALCOHOLIC

"I was angry all the time, out of control, ripping mad, alienating my friends, laying guilt on my kids, obsessing about his vacations with his girlfriend, about money, feeling like shit day and night."

LAURA, 42-YEAR-OLD RECENTLY DIVORCED

SELF-CONFRONTATION

Immersed in the immobilization stage, our first hurdle involves naming the problem and admitting fully to ourselves just how bad things really are. Easier said than done. It is rarely clear to us that we are not yet facing the situation directly.

We tend to mistake the obvious surface details for the source of our suffering and ignore the root cause. The impulse to rationalize one thing and make excuses for another protects us from the intensity of self-confrontation. One of the key factors that stands in the way is our degree of unreadiness to face ourselves head on. Often, we're just not ready to look at the whole picture.

And yet, as **Henry Miller** put it, "Everything we shut our eyes to, everything we run away from, everything we deny, denigrate, or despise, serves to defeat us in the end. What seems nasty, painful, evil, can become a source of beauty, joy, and strength, if faced with an open mind."

It is the nature of crisis to continue for durations in which the magnitude of the problem is not fully grasped. It is during such phases that our unconscious, unhelpful, or even destructive patterns are unwittingly perpetuated despite ongoing evidence that things are only getting worse. The longer we avoid facing the reality of the situation, the longer we remain trapped in place. Here in **Rainer Maria Rilke's** poem, *The Panther*, is a perfect description of this painful state.

> *His vision, from the constantly passing bars,*
> *has grown so weary that it cannot hold anything else.*
> *It seems to him there are a thousand bars;*
> *and behind the bars, no world.*
> *As he paces in cramped circles, over and over,*
> *the movement of his powerful soft strides*
> *is like a ritual dance around a center*
> *in which a mighty will stands paralyzed.*

Although our stories are different—betrayal, defeat, addiction, loss, injury, illness, etc.—this poem captures the essence of being painfully trapped, which is exactly how we feel when our life is out of control and we have no idea how to get it back on track. There is a fleeting glimpse, an impulse to break free, and then, arresting despair. These images are a precise metaphor for the emotional imprisonment of immobilization.

And our only way out of it is through it. Our first step out is to dig beneath the surface details to uncover our operating assumptions, the illusory ground on which we have been standing. To the extent that some of our basic premises are flawed—and we all have blind spots—there's a good chance that we are working on the wrong agenda, wearing ourselves down to no avail, confusing activity with progress, and basically going nowhere.

EXISTING MIND-SET

The key issue to address at this point is our preexisting mind-set, which determines our current take on the situation. Based on our initial operating premise, certain actions will seem perfectly logical, and other options will not even occur to us. Due to the subjectivity of all perception, our choices will fall within a limited range.

It is always hardest to be objective about our own issues. Stuck at an impasse, our tendency is to perseverate, repeating and redoubling our efforts, even though they have not proved effective so far, and, at the same time, ignoring alternative ways of looking at the situation.

Be honest. Where and when have you tried the same tactic over and over, only to experience frustration? Now is the time to examine your life in search of dead-end efforts. First let's look at your prevailing mind-set with regard to the crisis you're facing. Your existing level of conscious awareness is reflected in your current attitudes and approaches. It is directly related to your core beliefs, the premises and assumptions that you take to be givens. This is about becoming a good detective and including yourself in the investigation.

If you believe that being a loving wife guarantees that you will be cherished, it is inconceivable that you could be mistreated indefinitely, so why leave? If you believe that you're irreparably damaged, where would you get the energy to make an effort? If you think your life is permanently ruined, why bother getting sober? If you think you are likely to fail, why try? If you believe you have no right to be happy, how long do you remain in an abusive situation? Bottom line, if you believe your obstacles are insurmountable, they are; and if you believe you have no viable options, you don't.

Uncovering your existing mind-set is the first fork in the road, right along with admitting to yourself how bad things really are. Until now, how have you been attempting to fix the problem and make your life work? Now is the time for consciousness-raising, for becoming more aware of both your recurring thoughts and the specific behaviors that flow from them. Self-observation requires the ability to watch ourselves, without criticism or blame, long enough to see what is actually there. The goal here is not to critique but to simply observe our thoughts, attitudes, and actions with increasing objectivity.

It takes courage and compassion to look at ourselves with this level of honesty. Naturally we squirm away. Yes, the truth will set us free, eventually, but first it will make us suffer. This is where self-compassion comes in. Without it, what we see can be too hard to accept. Dread of being wrong or at fault—responsible for this mess we're in—works against us. We may end up feeling something we never wanted to feel. Resistance sets in and keeps us running in place.

There is a way out of the woods, however. It begins with becoming more skillful at calming your body, first through body awareness and then by releasing tension with the exhale. Until we develop this natural ability to intervene on our own behalf, to self-soothe, self-regulate, and then exercise choice, we remain spinning in place or frantically casting about, but more or less lost in space indefinitely. In an excerpt from *Lost,* poet **David Wagoner** speaks to the need for pausing and observing more and more keenly, as a practice.

> *Stand still. The trees ahead and bushes beside you*
> *Are not lost. Wherever you are is called Here,*
> *And you must treat it as a powerful stranger....*
> *No two trees are the same to Raven.*
> *No two branches are the same to Wren.*
> *If what a tree or a bush does is lost on you,*
> *You are surely lost. Stand still. The forest knows*
> *Where you are. You must let it find you.*

Self-observation is a crucial first step and the most effective catalyst to progress at this point. What are you saying to yourself, repeatedly? What emotions are you feeling as a consequence of that very thought? What actions are you then taking again and again? What is the hardest thing to admit to yourself? Take a moment, slow down, look at your life, and notice how you are right now. Just observe.

As the poem suggests, "If what a tree or bush does is lost on you, then you are truly lost." Now is the time to look, with a clear and courageous eye, at what's in front of you. It's about piercing through the buffer of your illusions and the comfort of your denial to reveal what's actually happening, to see it for what it is, and to identify your place in it.

SELF-OBSERVATION

Take a moment to consider the crisis you are facing:

- What is the worst part of this for you?
- What makes you saddest?
- What makes you angriest?
- What makes you most afraid?

Now comes the next significant challenge. The more we become self-observant, the more we need to deal with fear, the biggest impediment to progress at this point. This is the time to shed light on its impact so that we can work with it more skillfully. The harsh truth is often too painful to let in. Facing what this means to us is often too unnerving or perhaps even frightening. A key factor in determining how long we will remain immobilized now is simply our relative level of stress hardiness. Fortunately, this is a very workable problem.

How can we increase our resilience, and therefore our readiness, to move through this phase? We must first recognize that fear is distorting our perceptions. Fear will amplify some things and filter out others. Fear can make challenging obstacles appear insurmountable while, at the same time, it is discounting our innate strengths and screening out alternative possibilities.

Whether we're feeling rage, horror or despair, there is an underlying element of fear in all painful emotions. Remember, acute stress involves the perception of a threat or danger to our physical or psychological well-being and the perception that this danger is beyond our ability to control. Perception is the operative word. It is extremely helpful at this point to have a vivid grasp of the role that fear is playing in keeping us stuck in our personal mind trap for hours, days, weeks, months, years.

THE MIND-BODY MATRIX

This section deals with the physiology of stress. A working knowledge of the basics is so relevant to the process of moving forward that I urge you to give it careful study. It's a crash course in Mind-Body Medicine 101: How anxiety affects the body.

In a nutshell, *every emotion is affecting our physical body, for better or for worse, all the time.* The intense fear we experience is having a significant impact on both our physiology and our perception. In response to elevated anxiety, many changes are simultaneously taking place in the body, governed by our autonomic nervous system: increases in our heart rate, blood pressure, oxygen need, respiratory rate, adrenalin, perspiration, and blood glucose levels, etc.

A whole cascade of responses is flooding through our body: neuroendocrine, cardiovascular, musculoskeletal, and immunological. Our digestive tract limits blood supply to muscles, and our blood vessels constrict. Our somatic motor system swings into action, affecting neuromuscular changes: Muscular tension increases, jaws clench, the body braces for action. Our sympathetic nervous system shifts into high gear.

Here is where our clarity begins to diminish as mind-altering changes begin to distort our perceptions. The central nervous system has kicked in, compromising our emotional intelligence and lowering our cognitive functioning as well as our ability to self-regulate, exacerbating our emotional suffering, and bringing out the worst in us from a behavioral standpoint.

This is how anxiety affects all of us—*mentally and emotionally*:
- Perception is distorted and narrowed down.
- Memory becomes imprecise and diminished.
- Learning is impaired and even blocked temporarily.
- We assume a defensive stance.
- We have a tendency to either regress or perseverate.
- Our anticipation becomes overly negative.
- We have the impulse to either dominate or cave in.

This is precisely when we lose our objectivity, just when we need it most. The higher our anxiety level, the more our perception of reality will be distorted. Imagine looking at the same Rorschach ink blot while in a state of anxiety or depression versus when we are calm and cool? The responses would vary dramatically.

Our interpretations of what we're "seeing" right in front of us are not objective. We are in an altered state, operating under the influence of our prevailing emotions. We find ourselves perseverating, going through the same ineffective motions over and over despite their observable fruitlessness.

Why is it so important to be aware of these subtle and obvious changes? So, we can understand just how anxiety compromises our ability to function at our best in any situation, let alone a time of crisis. When stress sends us into flight, fight, freeze mode, we lose access to our full cognitive capacities. It's as if our functional IQ drops about 40 points and our body, flooded with stress hormones (adrenalin, noradrenalin, cortisol), produces physical sensations that often feel incapacitating. As our stress level goes up, our impulse control and ability to self-regulate behaviorally, go down.

Three key factors are involved in dis-regulating the physical body with regard to anxiety states: *intensity, frequency, and duration.* Given enough exposure, we eventually become susceptible to developing a whole range of stress-related medical problems that only complicate matters: chronic hyper-arousal, high blood pressure, arrhythmias, irritable bowel syndrome, fibromyalgia, sleep disorders, muscle spasms, chronic headaches, chronic back pain, metabolic and digestive disorders, allergies, neuromuscular problems, rashes, autoimmune problems, anxiety disorders, depression, cancer, and cardiovascular disease, to name a few.

The *good news* is that, once we're aware of how stress is affecting us, we can begin to work with it more skillfully. We can learn how to effectively manage our stress level in any and every difficult situation. We can develop our capacity to remain in command of ourselves no matter what. This is the goal, and it is achievable.

Remaining calm opens up the possibility of choice. And choice is crucial for change and growth. By enhancing our basic resilience, we become increasingly empowered to handle whatever difficulties come our way. Developing our stress hardiness is not only essential for moving through crisis, it is a spiritual strength and life skill that will serve us in every aspect of personal and public life going forward.

Self-command is the highest elegance.
RALPH WALDO EMERSON

EXERCISE: MINDFULNESS, BODY AWARENESS, AND THE RELEASE OF TENSION

To face challenge most effectively, we first need to learn how to focus on calming our physical body so that we can think with a full deck. The more skillful we become at releasing stress and tension, the more quickly we restore our body to a healthy state and our mind to full functioning. During this first phase of immobilization, we need to become more aware of the tension level in the body so that we can learn to work with it effectively.

Developing mindfulness is the first crucial step to expanding our basic conscious awareness. With increased body awareness, we become more keenly observant of our physiology, more conscious of our anxiety sensations early in the game, just as they begin to occur. The more present we become, the easier it is to track the feeling of tension arising in the body. The sooner we notice, the sooner we can use mind-body skills to intervene and release the tension.

The most direct and instantaneous way to lower your tension level is simply to notice and slow down your inhale and exhale. This powerful tool is invisible and free. Breathing deeply and fully with a soft belly will do more for your tension level than any gadget, gismo, mantra, or escape. We will build on this as we go on. But for now, the most effective way to proceed through the immobilization phase is to become adept at calming your physical body.

In purely clinical terms, we are eliciting the relaxation response by focusing on the breath while in a relaxed position, releasing tension with the exhale, and opening to the present moment. Even three to five breaths can effectively bring your anxiety down to a manageable level. Think of it: you are never more than three deep breaths away from feeling better, enough to regain some space from the issue at hand.

It's still just a beginning, but it is crucial to the process. By enhancing your ability to calm your body, and consequently your mind, you are in effect unlocking the prison door. You are no longer trapped, blocked, powerless, at the mercy of your negative thoughts and painful emotions. You are doing something constructive and helpful in this very moment. You are also learning how to enhance your emotional stamina and stress hardiness to your long-term benefit.

This is the first developmental task we will need to start working with. As long as our anxiety level is out of control, we will not make significant progress. More than likely, we will either remain roughly at a standstill, engaged in fruitless efforts, or we will actually regress. Yet this moment offers a pivotal opportunity for growth to happen. Why yield to fear, effectively abdicating your power to choose?

> *Whatever arises in your life*
> *is the right material*
> *to bring about your growth*
> *and the growth of those around you.*
> MARCUS AURELIUS (121-180 AD)

Assuming for now, or at least acknowledging the possibility, that somehow every hardship and adversity contains a special purpose or hidden blessing, take a slow deep in-breath, hold it for a few seconds, and then watch it turn into an exhale, releasing fully with the out-breath. Get into a comfortable position in a peaceful, safe place. Breathe in slowly and deeply, allowing your eyes to close and your muscles to soften and relax, inhaling the present moment right here and now, right in the midst of everything that is painful, frightening, and unresolved. Then exhale any tension you notice in the body, letting a natural restfulness wash over you and through you.

Beginning at the top of the head and scanning through the full length of your body, invite and allow each area to soften and relax. This is a moment of self-nurturing that only you can do for yourself. For now, just be aware of the sensations in the body as you scan through it, as if you were sweeping the body with your breath. Notice the length of every inhale and exhale, with particular emphasis on the exhale, and then see if you are able to slow it down a bit more.

Practicing this kind of focused breathing for even ten minutes twice a day can begin to have a profound effect on your ability to handle life's challenges. Now is the time to develop your ability to tolerate the turmoil ahead, to become more and more resilient, more and more able to meet the challenges, to grow in conscious awareness, equipped to transform your life, despite the seemingly impossible obstacles in your path.

STAGES AT A GLANCE

Summary Points for this chapter and those that follow, begin with a generic quote and cover the following experiential components associated with that stage:

Cognition [our current sense of what is happening]

Premise [our operating assumption or existing mindset]

Negative Automatic Thoughts [our recurring unhelpful thoughts]

Reasonable Realistic Response [a more rational statement than our NAT]

Emotions [how we feel psychologically while in this stage]

Physical [how our physiology is affected by those emotions]

Behavioral [how we tend to behave when this is going on]

Spiritual [how we are exeperiencing our situation spiritually]

Realization/Insight [what new insight is potentially available]

Catalysts and Impediments

    Potential pitfalls [risks for thwarting our progress]

    Catalysts to growth [skills for staying on track]

Exercise/Meditation [practices to support the process]

Poetic Images [poetic metaphors with which to connect]

Questions to Ponder [questions for opening and fortifying]

SUMMARY POINTS: PHASE I:
IMMOBILIZATION: BECOMING STUCK

"I am beside myself. I can't even think straight."
EXCERPT FROM CASE STUDY

Cognition: My life is a mess outside and inside; the pain is excruciating.

Premise: This can't be happening, should not be happening to me.

Negative Automatic Thought (NAT): I feel trapped, stuck, like a failure, like my life is over—an utter failure; this is killing me, I could die, I wish I were dead.

Emotions: elevated anxiety, sense of hopelessness, defeat, fear, outrage, sadness; feeling unloved, disregarded, rejected, alone, adrift, unimportant to anyone, alternately afraid, terrified, helpless, hopeless, stunned, numb

Physical: stress-related symptoms, including headaches, digestive problems, allergies, rashes, sleep issues, chronic pain, hyperactivity or lethargy, weight gain or loss, substance dependency

Behavioral: addictive tendencies and avoidance behaviors, pretending, shutting down, withdrawing, perseverating

Spiritual: denial, numbness, deadening

Realization/Insight: I'm out of control; my whole life is my problem.

Catalysts and Impediments

Potential pitfalls: staying here indefinitely, paralyzed by fear, rage, or denial; with a continually elevated stress level, blaming others, numbing out, being defensive, obsessive, compulsive, or in denial

Catalysts to growth: learning basic stress reduction skills: increasing body awareness, mindful breathing, practicing calming the body and mind; self-observation

Exercise/Meditation: Practice mindfulness, increase body awareness, and become skillful at eliciting the relaxation response: the release of tension.

Poetic images: The Panther, Lost

Questions to Ponder: How long would you like to remain in this phase before moving forward? Recognize that you hold the key.

CHAPTER 2

Unraveling—Breaking Down: Chaos

This chapter maps out the second phase, chaos, which involves the shattering of illusions, an unraveling of what and who we thought we were before the unstoppable crisis occurred. It involves our need to self-confront, to examine our life outside of previous contexts, challenge our basic assumptions, and become better at tolerating uncertainty. Stress-reduction skills are crucial to progress. Almost imperceptibly, we are moving forward. Unraveling is actually very good news.

And this is the simple truth: that to live is to feel oneself lost—
he who accepts it has already begun to find himself,
his authenticity, to be on firm ground.
Instinctively, as do the shipwrecked,
he will look around for something on which to cling,
and that tragic, ruthless glance, absolutely sincere,
because it is a question of saving himself,
will cause him to bring order into the chaos of his life.
These are the only genuine ideas:
the ideas of the shipwrecked.
All the rest is rhetoric, posturing, farce.
He who does not really feel himself lost,

is lost without help; that is to say,
he never finds himself,
never comes up against his own reality.
JOSÉ ORTEGA Y GASSET

SHIPWRECKED

During the second phase, we feel shipwrecked as we begin to experience the breaking down of life as we knew it. Our previous way of being starts to collapse into its inevitable unraveling. We see that our once adequate tools (our survival skills, management strategies, and defense mechanisms) have become increasingly ineffective. It feels chaotic and painful. But this is completely natural and potentially fruitful.

While our (controlling) impulse is often to hold on tighter to the turning wheel of life, this is precisely when we need to loosen our grip and begin to shift our relationship to this change that is clearly unstoppable. Inner chaos feels frightening, but it is neither a mistake nor a failure. It is a necessary and unavoidable part of the process.

From the ancient Taoist perspective, change is the dynamic essential nature of the universe. It feels like a shattering of life, and it is. But it is also part of the great mystery that we are entering into.

Life does not accommodate you, it shatters you.
It is meant to, and it couldn't do it better.
Every seed destroys its container
or else there would be no fruition.
FLORIDA SCOTT MAXWELL

Our long-held views, assumptions and beliefs — the ones that have been framing our perceptions until now—are no longer holding up. Now is the time to lift the veil and take a closer look at whatever is underneath because what is happening on the surface no longer makes sense to us.

Our previous way of managing and relating to ourselves, our loved ones, to life and/or to the world is clearly not working. There's a deep recognition that life, as we know it, will never be the same. We're in an abyss, experiencing a sense of turmoil, uncertainty, confusion, and instability. Denial, once held in place by an undercurrent of fear, is now giving way to despair. We feel lost and chaotic.

CHAOS

It is worth noting that the word chaos, which we now take to mean only confusion and disorder, meant something very positive in the original Greek derivative. In ancient Greece, although chaos was synonymous with chasm and abyss, it actually signified a sort of *creative nothingness.*

Chaos meant the infinity of space and formless matter that preceded the existence of the ordered universe, a state of nothingness, as opposed to the existence of life, or state of being. We now think of a chasm as an unbridgeable gap or breach; we think of an abyss as a bottomless pit or gulf. But in ancient cosmogony, nothingness [chasm, abyss] meant the primal chaos before creation. From time immemorial, this period of chaos has been seen as having a dignity and purpose of its own.

Why does this matter? Because if we perceive inner chaos only as a negative state, a mistake or defeat, as something to avoid or hurry out of, we will shortchange ourselves and miss the full potential it offers us. With chaos re-envisioned as a period that precedes creative emergence, we can actually welcome it as a good thing and become more accepting and pragmatic about our emotional pain. We can interpret chaos not as our miserable and depressing failure, but as an important opportunity for growth.

In this context, inner chaos can be regarded as natural, even mythic. It becomes something that we can work with consciously, digging deeply into it for the insights that we most need to uncover. From a Buddhist perspective, adversity is the raw material of indestructible happiness.

When met with mindfulness skills, adversity can be a conduit to eventually experiencing equanimity, an abiding sense of calm and resilience in the face of crisis. Breaking down is still painful, but it is far more tolerable once we understand what an important purpose it can serve in our life.

You must have chaos within you
in order to give birth to a dancing star
FRIEDRICH NIETZSCHE

How do we feel during the breaking down phase? Like a cork bobbing in the ocean. Like we're walking around with an inner chasm: a sense of disconnection within ourselves, a sense of moorlessness outside ourselves.

Sometimes we feel abysmally sad. We spend time fluctuating between denial and dread, apathy and despair, deteriorating but not caring, withdrawing and faking it. But at the same time, something new is also happening: We're beginning to face the issues. We are uncovering important truths just below the surface.

Yes, there are moments of feeling lost, feeling that our life is ruined. We still feel confusion, panic, horror, disgust, disbelief, loneliness, like we're going crazy, a sense of purposelessness and nothingness. Then there's the fear of becoming even more anxious and the fear that things will get even worse. This is how it feels and *exactly how it's supposed to feel* when things are breaking down. It means we are making progress. We are no longer frozen in place.

From the perspective of Buddhist psychology, our deepest emotional pain is the seed of our greatest potential freedom from emotional suffering—i.e., from our tendency to cycle indefinitely in chronic frustration and dissatisfaction. Crisis can serve as the most important and effective impetus to our transcending the habitual thinking patterns of our conditioned existence, as well as all the cultural influences that shape our perceptions to our detriment.

In this context, emotional pain can actually be embraced as an initiation into a higher level of consciousness on the path to liberation from the bondage of a more constricted way of being—*if* we work through it as such. It is all a matter of perspective.

How are we relating to what is happening? When philosopher and poet Kahlil Gibran said, "Your pain is the breaking of the shell that encloses your understanding,... the bitter potion by which the physician within you heals your sick self," he was echoing this insight. Sufi mystic **Kabir** reminds us, in this excerpt from ***The Time Before Death***, that now is the perfect time to do this work:

> *"If you do not break the ropes while you're alive,*
> *do you think ghosts will do it after?...*
> *The idea that the soul will join with the ecstatic*
> *just because the body is rotten—that is all fantasy.*
> *What is found now is found then...*
> *If you make love with the divine now, in the next life you*
> *will have the face of satisfied desire...*
>
> KABIR

As the Chinese character for *crisis* suggests, there is always both danger and opportunity within our difficulties, with the possibility of something new and better becoming available. From this perspective, crisis can be viewed as having an aspect of transformation inherent in it.

> *Chaos should be regarded as very good news.*
> CHOGYAM TRUNGPA RINPOCHE

There are three aspects to the chaotic breaking down phase. It begins with introspection and then questioning or challenging our working assumptions, the "givens" that we need to uncover. Actively engaging in these processes moves us forward toward the third aspect, our threshold. Now is the time to measure our woundedness and come clean to ourselves like it's our job, our sacred duty.

It's time to observe the fear that this brings up and to practice becoming calm in the face of it. It's time to practice choosing to trust the process of change. Again and again. I emphasize practice because that is what it takes to integrate what is for many of us a radically new way of being. Is it difficult to practice this? Of course. But it's nowhere near as difficult as going through life without these insights, tools, and newly established spiritual strengths.

As harrowing as it is, crisis provides experience that brings valuable insights that we might never grasp otherwise. Here's where the idea of crisis as opportunity comes in. However devastating the situation we're in, there remains the possibility of drawing something of tremendous value from it. Something that will serve ourselves and others. Something we could not have acquired any other way. Like the wild storm that knocks dead branches from the tree, leaving only the essential core, it is through crisis that we can encounter that which is indestructible in ourselves.

INTROSPECTION—FACING WHAT MUST BE FACED

LAURA'S STORY Laura had been stuck in an endless cycle of agonizing about the many painful realities of her life. Her ex-husband's heartless behavior toward her, his relationship with his girlfriend, her fears about her children's loyalty, and her nagging financial insecurity—these were the top four issues that kept her spinning all day and awake all night. The intensity of her outrage, jealousy, and fear was particularly troubling as it had already been four years since the divorce. All the "protest tears" in the world were obviously not moving her forward, as she continued to rail against the reality of her situation. She was inconsolable.

The prospect of remaining trapped in this painful pattern indefinitely was so frightening and depressing to her that it actually fueled her motivation to do the hard work of freeing herself. Laura became adept at relaxation skills in record time, learning to calm her body and mind through basic breathing techniques, described in the previous chapter. Once she was able to consistently calm her body, she progressed naturally into the next phase.

She was then able to honestly face the worst of it and eventually take the steps in moving forward by taking a closer look at her fears and beginning to investigate her pain at a deeper level. This meant stepping back and naming what was worst about her crisis, measuring its impact on her, and then feeling her feelings. All of them.

It has long been said that if you can feel it, you can heal it. Without some compelling justification, why would anyone one risk this further pain? But just as an infection beneath the skin surface must be lanced to allow drainage and facilitate healing, this is the time to lean into the pain and honestly face the worst of it so that it can gradually be released in ways that we will now explore.

The need for change
bulldozed a road down the center of my mind.
MAYA ANGELOU

We get the courage to do this only because we recognize that, until we shed more light on the root problem, key insights will remain hidden from us. "There can be progress only by shattering your understanding to allow a greater understanding to come through," Pir Vilayat Inayat Khan reminds us. The process of introspection is also the very springboard we need most to wake up to the full significance of what is present, here and now.

The goal is to uncover our deepest feelings and beliefs about ourselves within the context of what is happening in our life at this very moment. While only you can do this for yourself, you don't need to do this by yourself. There are many good ways to proceed, using important tools like reflection, meditation, and journaling, as well as working with a therapist and/or close friend, or spouse. There are always some hidden biases and unconscious beliefs inside of us that are running the show from behind the scene. Now is the time to uncover them, to face where our efforts have been fruitless, where we have remained spinning in place, and where we have repeatedly invested ourselves in unworkable options.

Emotional pain can serve a valuable purpose; it can even serve as a gateway to freedom, according to Buddhist psychology, which has made an invaluable contribution to Western thought.

Although human suffering is universal, crisis can be transformed into expansion, depending on how we work with it. Adversity can be harnessed as a catalyst to growth. It is only when our outmoded assumptions and premises break down that the possibility of something new and better becomes available.

From the Buddhist perspective, we will all eventually find ourselves immersed in the wheel of *samsara*, spinning off in the vicious cycles of our conditioned existence, our deeply ingrained attitudes, oblivious to our blind spots. We have been attempting to solve the unsolvable, using the very tools (our old ones) that unwittingly perpetuate our suffering. We have been operating within the limitations of a lower level of conscious awareness, trapped in habit patterns, feeding false hopes, yielding to fears, and reinforcing illusions with every unquestioned reaction.

No amount of raging to friends about her ex-husband's behavior or worrying about her financial issues every night had helped to move Laura forward and out of pain. She'd spent her energy either agonizing about her life or escaping from agonizing. When asked to investigate her anger, fear, and sadness more fully, she was naturally skeptical.

Going any deeper into her pain seemed counterintuitive, senseless, even risky. She could barely hold it together as it was. But she'd been learning to calm herself through body awareness and breathing techniques, and this had been empowering for Laura. It helped her proceed without fear of being overwhelmed. She was beginning to feel encouraged and hopeful for the first time in years.

Laura could now look directly at herself for a change—this time really seeing the state she had been in for so long and the negative impact it was having on her life. First, the physical toll on her health: digestive and sleep problems, the headaches, her skin breaking out, the weight gain. Then behaviorally: her inability to make healthy food choices and exercise regularly, extra glasses of wine, irritability at work, her short temper with the children. Then emotionally: her diminished self-worth, lagging energy and enthusiasm, jealousy toward her happily married friends, loneliness now, and, worse, her fear of being alone forever.

She realized she was beating herself up with the fantasy that her ex-husband, who had so mistreated her, had magically reformed into being a wonderful partner in his new relationship. Spiritually, she felt a pervasive sense of crisis and, worse, the groundless feeling that she was no longer intact. And yet, she was beginning to make progress.

It takes thorough inventory-taking and courageous self-confronting to move ourselves forward from the abyss. We need to face and acknowledge the full reality of precisely where we are right now. So Laura became "fierce with reality," as F.S. Maxwell has suggested. She made a key discovery: It was unmanaged stress and an inability to tolerate chaos that had been keeping her stuck in place so long. Once she became more adept at calming, self-soothing, lowering her anxiety level, she was then able to make progress.

Introspection is needed for damage assessment, for creating a full report on yourself, to yourself. First we lift the curtain of pain without backing away. Then we embrace everything we find with honesty and self-compassion. Yes, this is unnerving, especially when we have a sense of being in conflict with ourselves over values, meaning, and the givens, our operating assumptions. It's also a crucial step in the process.

Another term for this inner conflict is cognitive dissonance, which has long been recognized as one of the most powerful agents of change. It

impels us toward naming and re-ordering our priorities. This clarifying of
our values is essential to living consciously, with intention and awareness.
It calls us to ask courageous questions again and again. Some degree of
progress is always within reach. It just takes courage.

The breeze at dawn has secrets to tell you.
Don't go back to sleep.
You must ask for what you really want.
Don't go back to sleep.
People are going back and forth across the doorsill
where the two worlds touch.
The door is round and open.
Don't go back to sleep.

RUMI

The important thing to keep recognizing is that, for all the pain
involved in looking more deeply into the wound, there is a liberating
aspect to this process. It can be understood as the naturally dynamic and
fluctuating rhythm of all life, the Tao of change, of decay and birth, chaos
and order, despair and emergence. This is the shaky ground on which
our potential for evolutionary change ultimately becomes possible as the
beliefs, expectations, and assumptions that have played a role in our crisis
begin to break down. Some of our most firmly held assumptions were
destined to unravel to in any case. They were the premises and paradigms
of our earlier life, our first adulthood, that no longer fit the reality of who
and where we are today.

QUESTIONING—ASKING COURAGEOUS QUESTIONS

The tree that would grow to heaven
must send its roots to hell.

FRIEDRICH NIETZSCHE

This is a time of self-observation, self-confrontation, and self-compassion—a time for questioning everything and finding the courage to face the very things we would most like to avoid. We may not feel ready for change yet, but we know we really can't go on like this. Now is the time to get past focusing on questions like Why me? Why now? Why this? What next? How can I go on? How could he/she do this to me? What have I done to deserve this? How long will it take to be OK? When will I ever feel safe again? Who can I trust now? How can I be happy? Where can I go now? How could this be happening?

It's also time to get past pretending that it's not that bad or that it's getting better when we know in our heart of hearts that it's not. We are making progress from ruminating on, "I can't believe what's happened to me," to being able to say, "It happened; now what?"

As important as the previous questions were, it will take very different ones to move us forward from here. So we begin asking new questions, the ones we maybe haven't thought of and the deeper ones we've been avoiding.

What you ask is who you are
and what shapes our lives is
the questions we refuse to ask
or never think of asking.

SAM KEEN

EXERCISE: SEED QUESTIONS

- Who am I right now?
- What really matters most now?
- What else?
- What would I rather not face right now?
- What is the hardest thing for me to accept here?
- What emotions am I feeling?
- What did I used to believe?

- What do I believe now?
- What do I want to believe?
- What is true for me in this moment?

These are some of the seed questions to return to again and again in contemplation, through journaling, and in dialogue with a trusted therapist or ally. It's a matter of doing due diligence on yourself. The more accurate information we have about our inner truth, the better equipped we are to make conscious, constructive choices and do the next right thing. Remaining in denial about the nature of our core issues only perpetuates the pain without moving us forward. This is a time of penetrating the illusions we've been holding about ourselves and about others. It's a time of rolling back the stone and facing whatever there is to face on deeper and deeper levels.

> *Your vision will become clear only when*
> *you look into your heart.*
> *Who looks outside, dreams.*
> *Who looks inside, awakens.*
> CARL JUNG

We need to bring to consciousness anything and everything there is to see, including our inevitable blind spots. This often takes some help from trusted others. As *Goethe* reminds us,

> *None are so hopelessly enslaved*
> *as those who falsely believe they are free.*

So we commit ourselves to this process of self-inquiry, accepting the challenge as one more courageous step forward, not because we're feeling comfortable with this, but simply because we are so done with spinning in place, remaining stuck in the comfort zone of denial or blame. Or perhaps we have no interest in having to suffer through one more painful lesson learned the hard way. So we just do it. We dig deep.

Where you stumble ... there lies your treasure.
The very cave you were afraid to enter ...
turns out to be the source
of what you were looking for.
The damned thing that was so dreaded ...
has become the center.

JOSEPH CAMPBELL

Ideally, we will alternate our times of self-inquiry with moments of solitude and contemplation, keeping a sense of quiet like an open space inside our hearts. It takes a while for really important answers to rise to the surface anyway. They will come in their own time. For now, it's enough just to be practicing stillness and self-observation, learning to calm our body and mind, letting the questions be open-ended, and accepting the brokenness of the present without rushing to solidify our thoughts with premature conclusions that may not serve us as well or even be accurate.

It's a time for being intensely, patiently, humbly observant. It's about cultivating peace and trusting the process. Meanwhile, we are developing our ability to self-confront with increasing awareness and enhancing our ability to self-soothe through mind-body relaxation tools. The following passage from **T.S. Elliot** speaks eloquently to this state of mind when we are simply "not ready for thought."

I said to my soul, be still, and wait without hope,
for hope would be hope for the wrong thing;
wait without love, for love would be love of the wrong thing;
there is yet faith, but the faith and the love and the hope

> *are all in the waiting.*
> *Wait without thought, for you are not ready for thought:*
> *So the darkness shall be the light, and the stillness the dancing.*

The next series of questions are designed to help move us closer toward the threshold of change. They will also serve as ongoing ones, particularly while our old way of being is dying off and our new life is struggling to be born. Take some time to explore these and the first ten questions listed earlier in this chapter, either through writing in a journal or in dialogue. We proceed, doing this, because, as **D.H. Lawrence** has observed,

> *We've got to live, no matter how many skies have fallen.*

EXERCISE: PROBING MORE DEEPLY

Ten more seed questions
- Do I really believe in the possibility of change and growth?
- What is holding me back?
- What will happen if I do nothing?
- Who is steering the boat of my life?
- What is my biggest fear right now?
- How is my fear affecting me?
- What purpose is it serving?
- How is it getting in the way?
- What makes me angriest?
- How is my anger affecting me?
- What purpose is it serving?
- How is it getting in the way?
- What do I want for myself in this new moment?
- What is the point?

*And the time came when remaining tight inside the bud
became harder than the risk it took to bloom.*

ANAIS NIN

Although we're still far from where we need to go, we're a long way from
where we've been. Addressing the questions in the previous section has
helped to move us forward, gaining critical mass. In the process of exploring our thoughts and feelings, the sense of unraveling in the breaking
down phase has become a reality. Old pretenses and illusions are beginning to collapse as the chaos intensifies. This is a good thing. Remember,
this is the nothingness that precedes the creation of a whole new order.

Some things are already different. We're in crash-and-burn mode one
minute and curiously calm in the next. New painful realizations keep
coming, but, more and more, we see ourselves taking them in stride, particularly if we are becoming adept at stress-reduction skills. The more we
practice, the better it works. Even three to five deep breaths can bring
about the shift we need in order to refocus. Our increasing ability to
manage our anxiety level and restore calmness in our body creates an
ideal inner environment for growth.

*Fear not the strangeness you feel.
The future must enter you long before it happens.
Just wait for the birth, for the hour of new clarity.*

RAINER MARIA RILKE

TED'S STORY It was during the breaking down phase that Ted began to
see that, no matter what the hardships were, he could no longer continue
at the engineering company he had managed so successfully for the last 16
years. An unusually good-natured and capable man, he had kept his nega-

tive feelings bottled up inside, smiling on the outside, withering on the inside. Yes, he had hated his work for easily 10 years, but the prospect of launching a new career, wasting his training and experience, and subjecting his family to financial risks seemed overwhelming. In a word, paralyzing.

He consistently dismissed the idea that making a change was a feasible consideration. After years of disregarding his true feelings, Ted realized that his physical and emotional well-being had become compromised. Headaches, psoriasis, sleeping issues, and mild depression had been steadily increasing his risk for serious chronic illness. His unhealthy lifestyle was one of overwork and feeling over-exhausted, with no energy and little time for joy in his life.

He initially sought therapy to learn stress-reduction skills so that he could increase his strength and cope with his unhappiness more effectively. Ironically, he was already too strong for his own good; he had been tolerating the intolerable to his own detriment. Once he began to fully acknowledge his sadness and inquire more deeply within himself, it became clear that he was in a far bigger crisis than he'd ever realized.

Despite his intelligence, capabilities, and talents, Ted secretly felt resentful, despairing, and strangely powerless. He could barely remember how happy, funny, vibrant, and alive he had once been. It took huge courage for Ted to ask himself the hard questions. He knew instinctively that, once he answered them, there would be no turning back.

Ted had always been able to rationalize his decision to stay with the game plan despite all the negatives. He'd thought he was indestructible, that he had to be the one to shoulder all of the responsibility. Fear of financial insecurity and marital pressure had locked him into a track that seemingly had no exit. The fact that he felt trapped and unhappy was irrelevant to everyone but Ted. But, step by step, he made his way through the phases, transitioning into a way of life that was better than he'd hoped for. Although the journey was never easy, it proved to be rife with challenges, discoveries, and wonderful rewards.

We are all faced with a series of great opportunities—
brilliantly disguised as insoluble problems.

JOHN GARDNER

Asking new and courageous questions initiated the first shift for Ted. What came into focus for the first time was realizing that his admirable sense of responsibility had gradually crossed the line into self-betrayal. Having a capacity for self-sacrifice is obviously a good thing, but, taken to an extreme, it ceases to be a virtue and becomes emotionally and physically unhealthy.

"This [my life] can only work when I'm not being true to myself on a very deep level. How did I get to this place? Whatever it takes, I just can't do this anymore. I am dying inside. I have to save myself." These were Ted's first frightening realizations, followed by "I don't want to be afraid anymore." And "My life matters too, doesn't it? Shouldn't it?"

The notion that he actually had a right to choose work that was fulfilling, even if it meant a major salary decrease, did not come easily to Ted. Seeing this issue as a healthy need was by no means a given. His deeply ingrained belief was that to make such a choice was reprehensibly selfish. This flawed but unquestioned premise had kept him tied in knots for years. His first steps forward were actually terrifying, although fear of failure was not the biggest obstacle. He was confident in his abilities for every good reason.

As it turned out, Ted's hidden immobilizing fear was that, if he did make this change, he would actually risk loosing what mattered most: He might no longer be loved; he might be despised and even abandoned, which was too humiliating and frightening to even imagine. Initially, he was completely unaware of these feelings, although they were just below the surface. But once he brought this fear to consciousness where he could work with it, reappraise it, and challenge its validity, his feeling of apathy was replaced with a growing sense of optimism and curiosity about the tasks ahead.

Next, he uncovered the false assumptions and limiting beliefs on which his fear had been based, and he began to explore them in therapy. He proceeded to release himself from the grips of these cognitive and emotional restrictions quite naturally within a very reasonable period of time. Ted still had to grapple with unknowns. But he felt curiously liberated, experiencing a sense of vitality and enthusiasm that he had not felt in years.

With a budding sense of self-loyalty, he proceeded through challenges ahead with unexpected energy. Whatever the sacrifices, it was all worth it because he knew he was looking forward to every day. He stepped into the mystery of his own life, opening to discoveries and unanticipated outcomes. He made friends with uncertainty, knowing in his bones that he was on the right track. It would take many efforts and iterations before Ted would arrive at his first major breakthrough, but he was moving forward; and that felt better than okay. He was no longer being held hostage by fear.

FLEAS AND CEILINGS   True, in Ted's case, the box he was in had been nailed shut by an unrecognized fear. But what about the box itself? How did he allow that to happen? How do any of us end up gasping for life in such a cramped and confining space?

That is a complex question, but certainly the arresting images that we have acquired in our conditioning play a big role in shaping our lives. Words of criticism in childhood can tyrannize us from behind the scenes, filtering out choices and narrowing our options. We probably have not wondered how fleas are trained to obey and perform in a flea circus, but it's actually quite relevant.

Fleas are born with the ability to jump more than 150 times their height, about 12 inches. To tame the fleas, trainers placed them in a four-inch jar with a lid on it. The fleas try very hard to jump high at first, banging up against the lid, bruising their heads. After only three days in the jar, they totally give up: They learn it is pointless to try, and they just stop trying.

Even when the lid is removed, they will not jump up. In fact, they will never jump higher than the four-inch level set by the lid. Their behavior is now set for the rest of their lives. They have been trained to operate within this arbitrarily imposed limitation, permanently. It's a form of learned helplessness. Powerlessness! They have literally forgotten who they are.

As long as we are not using our full potential, we may as well not have it, because as far as our future is concerned, we no longer do. It is true that "Life shrinks or expands in proportion to one's courage," as Anais Nin suggests. But it is rarely that simple. Limiting factors include more than just lack of courage. There is also the undercurrent of despair that comes with any form of learned helplessness or conditioned powerlessness. This must first be identified and overcome in order to recover innate powers and gifts that have been forgotten along the way.

THRESHOLD QUESTIONS

- What were you like during the most confident, triumphant moments of your life?
- In your very best vision of yourself, how would you see yourself dealing with your challenges right now?

> *You must give birth to your images.*
> *They are the future waiting to be born.*
> RAINER MARIA RILKE

The chaos of the breaking down phase begins to acquire a whole new flavor as we now approach the threshold. Even in the most broken moments, there are times when the true self begins to reveal itself, like a bright shining star that's come out during the darkest night. And we've become more and more able to remain present in the midst of the harrowing confusion and imperfection of our life, without yielding to fear and withdrawing into regressive patterns of the past.

It's enormously important to be receiving some compassion and unconditional positive regard from supportive helpers, friends, and loved ones during this time. But we can't always count on that kind of support. The only consistent solution can be found within. Radically new levels of self-acceptance and inner befriending are needed. And these must come forth gradually and naturally from deep inside.

You have to accept whatever comes
and the only important thing is that
you meet it with the best you have to give.
ELEANOR ROOSEVELT

The more we immerse ourselves in the experience of transformation, the more we come to realize that it is an ongoing, natural process available to everyone who is genuinely seeking it. Every moment of our life is a bifurcation point, a fork in the road, a matter of choice. Every moment is an opportunity for waking up or for dreaming. In every crisis of every ordinary day, a stunning array of possibilities are offered to us. Every repeated choice determines which of our different tendencies we are presently grooving and reinforcing. Every action has an impact, for better or for worse. Each choice can serve to either constrict or expand our conscious awareness, on a moment-to-moment basis. It is in exercising our power to choose that we determine who we are and who we are becoming.

Although from the outside it may seem that suffering is pervasive during the breaking down phase, the fact is that we can always, at any moment, step into the present with mindfulness, creating space within. We can pause, breathe, reflect, and choose to release a negative thought, once we identify it. By contrast, when we are lost in our fears, withdrawing into old habit patterns of spinning out and shutting down, we simply do not see that we even have choices.

Our limited perspective creates a confirmation bias against seeing all that is actually there. Instead we tend to perceive what we are expecting to perceive. We unwittingly seek evidence that confirms our preset notions while we reject contradictory evidence. We are oblivious to the fact that our inner software has some serious bugs and that our freedom of choice is severely compromised by old tapes playing inside our heads. We've lost our autonomy and our perspective. We've been looking at the night sky through a straw.

> *I wake from sleep and take my waking slow.*
> *I learn by going where I need to go.*
> THEODORE ROETHKE

We always do have a choice about how we will relate to what is happening in any and all circumstances, moment to moment, breath by breath. It's about remembering that we have a choice and then just exploring it. As Mark Twain noted, "The man who does not read good books has no advantage over the man who cannot read them." If we do not exercise our power to choose, we have no advantage over someone who truly has no choice. To what extent is a life of limitation and "quiet desperation," as Henry David Thoreau calls it, an abdication of our innate power to choose?

These excerpts from *The Journey*, by **Mary Oliver**, speak to the experience of finally coming to grips with the crumbling hold of the past and the emergence of one's authentic voice, if only a whisper at first.

> *One day you finally knew*
> *what you had to do, and began.*
> *... the stars began to burn*
> *through the sheets of clouds,*
> *and there was a new voice*
> *which you slowly*
> *recognized as your own.*

One of the priceless gifts of the breaking down phase, for all its painful disillusionment, is the realization that only we can save ourselves, as Mary Oliver suggests later in her poem, *The Journey*: "Determined to do the only thing you could do—determined to save the only life you can save." The sooner we accept that harsh reality, the better. No one can do this for us, and no one can spare us this arduous developmental task. Going through life like a well-trained flea is always an option. Or we can choose to uncover and overcome the obstacles to our own unfolding. We are not genuinely alive just because we are not clinically dead.

We can work at removing the emotional hooks that keep us psychically anchored to painful situations and deadening mind-sets. In fact, this is the way forward. Because *no one else can destroy us, and no one else can save us.* No one has that power over us unless we give it to them. We are now at a crossroad, moving toward a threshold for change. Take your time. Questioning our beliefs, exploring our fears (conscious and unconscious), challenging our premises and assumptions for flaws and inaccuracies—all of this helps move up through the paradigmatic myopia of old ways and into the light of a new day.

NEUROPLASTICITY

There has never been more compelling evidence that we are wired for change. Current research in neuroscience unequivocally confirms that, thanks to our body's inherent neuroplasticity, our brains are continuously morphing and reconfiguring in response to our repeated activities and thoughts. We become what we practice being, not just metaphorically, but from the standpoint of body, mind, spirit, psyche, and subtle energy. Worry constantly, and we become a gold medalist at worrying. Every time we practice letting go and calming ourselves in the midst of a stressful moment, we become more adept at doing so the next time. Eventually, this stress-hardiness skill becomes second nature to us as a newly established and dependable trait.

If we have been practicing relaxation skills, increasing awareness of tension in our body, slowing down our breathing, and becoming more adept at releasing the tension., we are beginning to notice that, even though there are still many factors causing us to feel emotionally distraught, we are catching it sooner. We are seeing how a thought begins in our mind, converts into an emotional state, and is immediately felt in the body as a physiological change.

This impact occurs continuously, but whether we are promoting wellness or getting worn down is up to us. Unpreventable stress will come to us in one form or another as long as we live. How we respond to it makes all the difference. How long we stay stressed is something else we can work with. The goal is to experience a quicker recovery of our mental equilibrium and physical homeostasis, promoting improved function on every level of existence—physical, cognitive, emotional, behavioral, and spiritual.

Every time we stop, breathe deeply, and reflect on how we are relating to what's happening right now, we interrupt old cycles of reactive behavior. We begin to see that we have options. Whatever is the most helpful, constructive next step, be it problem solving or an emotion-focused strategy, we have created a tiny but a pivotal space in which the possibility of choice becomes available. Mindless perseverating keeps us stuck. Mindful awareness opens us to choice. Instead of fight or flight, we are consciously choosing light. This is about self-mastery.

Self-command is the highest elegance.
HENRY DAVID THOREAU

There's a famous teaching story about three Indians walking home one night and suddenly seeing a deadly cobra lurking at them from the side of the road. One man screams and runs; his reaction was flight. The other futilely tries to stone the cobra to death; his reaction was fight. The third man responds by calmly striking a match and seeing that it is merely a fallen branch shaped like a snake. He has chosen light. Things are rarely as they seem when seen through the eyes of fear.

Every time we practice relaxation skills and consistently calm ourselves, we are actively participating in our own transformation in ways we've only recently come to appreciate. As resilience and stress-hardiness develops through mindful awareness and focused breathing, we become increasingly able to handle situations and experiences that were previously too uncomfortable for us to tolerate. This explains our past tendencies to deny, escape, regress, withdraw, lash out, shut down, etc., when things got difficult. Increasing our emotional stamina has massive implications for improving our inner life as well as our relationships across the board.

As we consider our intention to make significant changes along with the anxiety this change generates, it is reassuring to know that our brain will be reshaping itself in response to our repeated efforts. As neuroscience has now demonstrated, when we are in the process of establishing a new habit, neural networks supporting the continuation of that chosen habit change accordingly, meeting us halfway in a sense. The expression "re-fire to re-wire" is absolutely true.

Not only are we built to manage change effectively, we can grow stronger and actually thrive in response to it. In fact, rather than attempting to organize our life in avoidance of change, there is a compelling argument for purposefully choosing change as a way of life. Psychologist and philosopher Erich Fromm taught that the secret of a creative and fulfilling existence was to regard the whole process of life as a process of giving birth, never taking any stage to be the final stage. **Abraham Maslow**, grandfather of the **Self-Actualization** and **Positive Psychology** movement wholeheartedly agreed:

> *We have, all of us, an impulse toward actualizing more of our potentialities toward self-actualization, or full humanness or*

human fulfillment ... This is a push toward the establishment of the fully evolved and authentic self ... an increased emphasis on the role of integration or unity, wholeness. Resolving a dichotomy into a higher, more inclusive unity amounts to healing a split in the person and making him more unified. This is also an impulse to be the best, the very best you are capable of becoming.

And then Maslow added this warning:

If you deliberately plan to be less than you are capable of being, then I warn you that you will be deeply unhappy for the rest of your life.

Now is the time to dig deep into our own being where layers and layers of conditioning and enculturation have shaped and influenced our perceptions. We all have hidden biases and limiting beliefs that we take to be real. What do you believe right now that might actually be false? What givens" and premises would you be willing to challenge?

What is key here is to acknowledge that we all do have some blind spots and flawed assumptions and then, with a certain humble curiosity and courageous discernment, maintain an open stance as we uncover them over time. As many wise people have noted, the true value of work is not what we get from it but rather what we become in the process of doing it. Nothing could be truer of the spiritual work involved in breaking down, breaking open, and breaking through.

Opportunities to find deeper powers within ourselves often come to us when life seems most challenging.
JOSEPH CAMPBELL

EXERCISE: MIND-BODY-SPIRIT QUESTIONS

- What contexts or conditions would be conducive for you to open your heart and mind to your best intuition, wisdom, insight?
- Where in your body do you need to relax your armor in order to receive?
- Where in your body can you relax constriction and tightness, allowing the blocks to dissolve on their own and allowing healing energy to flow freely in your body and in your life?
- Where in your spirit can you express and release holding of old pain, old stagnant energy that has been held in your physical and emotional body for so long: the fears, the resentments, the losses, the heartaches?
- And most importantly, why does it matter?

In conclusion, the breaking down phase is actually a good thing, an essential part of the process, though it may feel like it is out of control. Whenever our natural impulse toward growth is thwarted by our fear-based impulse to maintain the status quo, we find ourselves at a standstill. We then delay the process of unraveling by attempting to exert control and prevent change. We often have the capacity to envision a better way, but not the capacity to act on it just yet. Fine.

At this point, self-observation is all that is needed; self-awareness paves the way. Readiness is then the gatekeeper of our progress. And the good news is that readiness can also be purposefully enhanced. Practicing stress-reduction skills, mindfulness, and body awareness will increase our ability stay calm enough to stay on track. Trust the process. As our stress hardiness grows, progress will become increasingly possible. The more we learn to calm our body and mind, the sooner we will move forward.

Bear in mind that there is a serious personal downside to remaining stuck in unresolved conflict indefinitely. We can withstand elevated anxiety levels for just so long before health problems begin to develop. From a purely mind-body standpoint, the potential pitfalls of not moving forward include physiological stress, loss of drive and enthusiasm, chronic anxiety and depression, susceptibility to genetic predispositions, suppressed immune function, skin problems, increased risk of cardiovascular disease, irritable bowel syndrome, allergies, and psychological exhaustion.

This is not surprising when we consider that every thought and every emotion is affecting us for better or for worse all the time. There is an open door between our psychology and our physiology. During the breakdown phase, the need for change brings a sense of unease, making us more susceptible over time to dis-ease. But we are equipped to face these challenges with better insights and tools. Increased awareness, self-inquiry, stress-reduction skills, emotional stamina and self-loyalty all work synergistically to help carry us out of the woods and forward, through the chaos.

> *In times of change, the learners will inherit the Earth*
> *while those attached to their old certainties*
> *will find themselves beautifully equipped*
> *to deal with a world that no longer exists.*
> ERIC HOFFER

SUMMARY POINTS: PHASE 2:
UNRAVELING—BREAKING DOWN

"This is a such a nightmare ... it's unbearable,
incomprehensible, insane"
EXCERPT FROM CASE STUDY

Cognition: This is happening, and it's even worse than I could have imagined. I'm beginning to see things differently.

Premise: I don't deserve this punishment; it's a terrible mistake.

NAT: Everything's broken, crumbling. My life is out of control. I am broken. Where or how I will end up: all alone? unloved? in constant pain? Something's got to give.

Emotions: instability and emotional intensity—waking up to fear, sadness, anger, humiliation, shame, groping, a sense of powerlessness

Physical: stress-related symptoms: headaches, rashes, insomnia, IBS, etc.

Behavioral: fluctuating between facing and denial/avoiding, more awareness during addictive and compulsive behavior, less escaping, the beginning of self-confronting and seeing the self differently; the need to receive emotional support

Spiritual: pervasive sense of crisis, chaotic, groundless, groping, feeling not intact, the unraveling of what was once intact

Realization: The dream (of how my life would be) is shattering, unpreventably. Illusions are collapsing. Change is unstoppable now. There is deep inner conflict: wanting change now but not being ready for it.

Catalysts and Impediments:

Potential pitfalls: blind spots, Achilles heel, flawed premises, hidden biases, unmanaged stress; the lack of a trusted, supportive ally; being stuck in a blame cycle

Catalysts to growth: Courageous questions; continuing self-inquiry and reevaluation: What have I been doing to avoid facing the reality of this situation? What previous reality (premise, assumption) no longer exists? Supportive relationships and the increasing ability to tolerate insecurity through mindfulness and stress-reduction skills

Exercise/Meditation: The focus is on self-inquiry; acknowledging reality as it is. This is okay. You must have a breakdown in order to have a breakthrough.

CHAPTER 3

Surrendering—Breaking Open

This chapter uncovers the third phase, surrendering, breaking open into the void that follows the collapse of our unsustainable defenses and illusions. It involves the need to soften, to loosen the grip of control as we reluctantly let go of past strategies, see and acknowledge where we are, and accept being with the painful reality, just as it is. New skills and strengths increase our receptivity to key insights and enhance our ability to navigate forward until the light gradually dawns.

"I really thought if something like this ever happened to me,
I would just die. But it all happened. And it didn't kill me"
EXCERPT FROM CASE STUDY

CULTIVATING A SENSE OF SURRENDER

As we move through the breaking down phase to begin the process of breaking open, cultivating a sense of surrender becomes very important. What comes to mind when you hear the word surrender? For many of us it has only a negative connotation: It means giving up, being defeated, losing a battle. But a certain quality of surrender is also an essential aspect of transformation. In fact, it is the next step.

Our prior way of being has been collapsing, unraveling, and disintegrating during the breaking down phase. Our mind and body feel like an inner combat zone. Our spirit is broken and chaotic. That is our current reality, our inner truth of the moment. We've asked the hard questions, felt our outrage, sadness, and fear. Our mind wants to go over it again and again because what has happened, or is happening, seems like such a mistake. It is so unacceptable, beyond our control, senseless, and all wrong.

But at some point there is simply nothing more to get from rehashing the details. Ruminating serves no purpose except to wear us down and keep us spinning in place.

PURPOSEFUL SOFTENING

Surrendering to the reality we are facing is actually a radical act. It is the most courageous and constructive thing we can possibly do. There's a part of us (our ego) that keeps clinging to the story of how things should have been, how we wanted our life to be, and perhaps what we have every right to deserve. It wants no part of accepting the reality of how it actually is. But no amount of resistance or refusal changes that fact. As **Flannery O'Connor** pointed out, *"Reality does not change according to our ability to stomach it."* After a while, all the gut-wrenching, hand-wringing, and protest tears in the world offer no consolation. They only perpetuate our misery.

Of course we all know this. But we don't want to know it. We have the illusion that by staying angry we are somehow memorializing the importance of how we have been wronged—by him or her or by the system or fate. We misconstrue this as self-loyalty. To simply let it go seems out of the question, as if that would mean trivializing the magnitude of our suffering.

There is this unconscious tendency to hold onto the pain with an iron grip. **Annie Dillard** once described how a ferret had sunk his teeth into the wing of a huge eagle that proceeded to fly away with the little ferret dangling from his wing. Rather than release the grip, the ferret starved to death with his jaws locked on the wing. He could have just let it go and survived.

Staying in denial (of how hurt we really are) is also tempting at this point, but equally unproductive. Pretending it's not that bad allows us to avoid facing our most uncomfortable feelings, providing a short-term fix for which we pay a long-term price. The protective wall we build around our heart also shields out the light, the joy, and the loving healing energy that we might otherwise be experiencing.

Encapsulated in denial, we have rendered ourselves unavailable to either the bad or the good. We end up cut off from ourselves and from others, emotionally, spiritually, and energetically, with our unprocessed pain shadowing us indefinitely and sapping our joy in the present. It's like having a chronic case of psychic indigestion from a gut full of un-metabolized emotional debris. By contrast—again, this takes some courage—we can investigate our pain with mindfulness and choose to view surrender as a rite of passage. Instead of running from our pain, we have a logical and valid reason to actually embrace it. This is an act of courage, in essence.

The practice of mindfulness, in this context, involves witnessing our most intense emotional states (of anger, sadness, fear) while cultivating a sense of calm through steady focused breathing, as described in the chapter discussing the mind-body connection. In doing so, we are increasing our physical and emotional resilience by the minute. The practice of deep steady breathing will naturally lower our anxiety level and restore physical equilibrium. This, in turn, allows greater access to our most objective and intelligent thinking. Our full cognitive ability returns.

It's only when we are physically and emotionally calmer that we can have the clarity to acknowledge and accept what must be acknowledged and accepted, that is, whatever the impossible reality actually is. This means saying, "It is what it is," and then consciously softening into it. And here is why. Surrender catalyzes the process of shifting from a state of unresolved conflict toward an inner ceasefire. This is the calm after the storm, bringing its own sense of peace.

When it seems humanly impossible to do more
in a difficult situation,
surrender yourself to the inner silence
and thereafter wait for
a sign of obvious guidance or
for a renewal of inner strength.

PAUL BRUNTON

Surrender carries us out of the breaking down phase and into the light of day, where breaking open becomes possible. But it is not a given. The ability to surrender also requires a temporary relinquishment of control, which certainly seems counterintuitive. In the face of anger and fear, our first impulse is to exert more control, not less. Yet from the perspective of both the individuals and the psychologists interviewed in my research (as well as so many poets and philosophers), our *ability to surrender* is emphasized as a crucial factor in the process of evolving.

For many of those who did triumph, it was during the surrender phase that they experienced a turning point—an unexpected thought, dream, or impulse that made all the difference in moving them into a new direction. Seemingly out of the blue, in the midst of intense surrendering, they felt the gridlock dissolving and got the first glimpse of a new idea or image that helped carry them forward. The critical hunch often seemed random at the time, but its significance became clear in retrospect.

We have the experience of softening into our painful reality, of allowing it to be what it is, followed by the sense of breaking open into new and fertile ground where some free space exists for an intervening impulse to occur. Resistance to reality blocks progress. Becoming more aware of exactly where our resistance is coming from is the first step in working with it consciously. There's a teaching from the Buddhist tradition that speaks directly to this: *Pain x Resistance = Suffering*. While pain is inevitable, the length and depth of our suffering will depend on our degree of resistance to what has already happened and cannot be undone no matter how fiercely we agonize, protest, or push against it. We can't un-ring the bell.

Sadly, we are capable of cycling in our suffering for years on end with the illusion that we really have no choice but to suffer, now that this pain has been inflicted on us by others or external circumstances. But again, it's not what *gets* us down, it's what *keeps* us down that matters in the end. And only we have the power to take the next step. Only you can unclench your fist.

When it comes to releasing ourselves from lingering emotional suffering, the following Rumi poem could not say it better.

> *I have lived on the lip of insanity,*
> *wanting to know reasons,*
> *knocking on a door. It opens.*
> *I've been knocking from the inside.*
>
> RUMI

This next step of surrendering is unlike all others, however. It is a step into the groundlessness of the present, where the past has been shattered and the future remains uncertain. It is the pause and the still point that precedes real change. It has been called the dark night of the soul, the ashes from which the phoenix emerges, etc. Surrendering is something we consciously *allow ourselves* to do. It cannot be forced.

Sometimes we surrender out of sheer exhaustion, having tried everything in vain to fix the unfixable. We are inconsolable. Our usual defenses are not cutting through the anguish. And we see that now there is nothing left to do to stop the war inside, but to disarm. This means we choose to acknowledge the pain and begin to soften into it. We begin to let it go. We begin to die to the past so that we can enter the present. This is what it's like to purposefully soften into it:

Being willing to sit in the dark,
being willing to not know,
to be terrified and to keep on sitting and letting go—
first of the not knowing, then of the terror,
then of all that you would cling to, letting go,
seeing it all as clouds blowing across the vast,
open sky, empty in and of itself.

CHINA GALLAND

Authentic transformation involves a death to the old self—to old beliefs, premises, and assumptions that have unraveled on their own—as a prerequisite for growing into our new self. We grow out of our old self not because it is easy to do, but because it becomes impossibly uncomfortable to remain within the confines of our previous way of being. Something's got to give. We can always try diminishing ourselves to fit inside a limited existence, as many people do.

Or we can shed this restrictive skin and grow forth. As **Kahlil Gibran** described in *The Prophet*, "Your pain is the breaking of the shell that encloses your understanding. Even as the stone of the fruit must break, that its heart may stand in the sun, so must you know pain." This is also part of the journey toward wholeness that Jung talked about. It is how we progress beyond the rules of our first adulthood to the individuation and autonomy of our second adulthood, as discussed earlier. To remain compliantly within the confines of our old shell is safe but ultimately suffocating.

EGO-CIDE

Jungian psychiatrist **David Rosen** explores this concept of breaking open in his book, *Transforming Depression: Healing the Soul through Creativity*. According to Rosen, at the core of the transformation process, is an archetypal death-rebirth experience, which he has termed **ego-cide**. Our ego (our conscious identity) is seen as a complex based on our personal history; it is a mix of personal unconscious and interjected parental characteristics and conflicts. If we are unaware of this complex and/or do nothing about it, we can remain merely an unconscious manifestation of our parental and cultural influences, limited by fears and restrictions that need to be outgrown, also known as the first adulthood.

"The Self is the force behind the sacrifice (symbolic death) of the dominant ego-image that is impeding individuation," says Rosen. We can only evolve to our true self through a *series of ego-cides*. This is how we free ourselves from what keeps us mind-trapped in old negative emotions. This is how we liberate and extricate ourselves from whatever tyrannizes and oppresses us. Only in dying to our old way of being can we be transformed into who we can become, discover our true purpose, and fulfill our personal myth and destiny. It's as if the decay and death of the old self serves as compost for the emergence of the true self; but until it dies off, the birthing is delayed.

Among the professionals interviewed in my research, "dark night of the soul" was defined as a universal experience involving major loss, despair, change beyond our control, acute crisis, devastating change, etc. There is a sense of being in grave danger and a realization that our defenses are crumbling under intense pressure from the impact of something much greater than our ability to hold at bay. A unanimous insight of these experts was that transformation is a very messy process: Profound change does not happen in a comfortable way, nor can it be forced according to some time or space. Yet transformative change clearly can be invited, cultivated, and even facilitated.

The dark night of the soul is
about the spiritual value of suffering
and the stripping away
of everything we have ever believed and relied upon.
MIRABAI STARR

THE OPENING

The breaking open stage of transformation seems to emerge spontaneously within the process of surrendering. *"You can't have a breakthrough
without a breakdown,"* as psychiatrist Alexander Lowen, MD put it. The
professionals interviewed in my research echoed this sentiment repeatedly.
Transformation occurs in the midst of darkness, chaos, and lack of control
of the situation. It only happens to individuals who are willing to temporarily tolerate these painful, sometimes terrifying, states and ride with them.

The good news is that we are hard wired for change and for transformation to happen, once we allow our resistance (to reality) to melt,
remaining present and mindful with exactly what is here at the moment,
however unacceptable that may be. We are moving toward fully facing
what we least wanted to face. This is the time for softening, for surrendering to what is, being with the reality of the situation, making friends with
uncertainty, and cultivating patience with this time of nothingness—and
for choosing to trust the process again and again. What if all you have to
do is be still and take time to be open and receptive to what is within you,
waiting to be revealed? Perhaps some strange, unanticipated blessing is
about to be realized. What if all you really need in the end is already deep
within you, waiting to unfold?

LETTING GO

Because all forms of resisting reality can only fail, it's time to soften into
what is, to give ourselves permission to finally surrender to it. This is
what it means to consciously work with the adversity we are facing. It
requires that we allow our shield of resistance to dissolve so that we can
begin to move forward. It's a little like passive solar. Simply by letting resistance go and cultivating inner silence, we are preparing the open space
for transformation to happen. Eventually, the light shows up and begins
to work for us.

Now is the time to become better and better at letting go of unrealistic expectations that will never be met, of prior strategies that have already failed, and of rigid demands that we have unwittingly placed on ourselves and others. Letting go can also mean unlearning, i.e., debriefing from old assumptions that either no longer support us or have already collapsed on their own. Sometimes, what is there to do but to be? And to trust that our painful emotions will undergo yet another shift once we allow them to soften as we practice letting them go. This excerpt from Mary Oliver's poem In Backwater Woods, captures this universal experience exquisitely.

> *To live in this world*
> *you must be able*
> *to do three things:*
> *to love what is mortal;*
> *to hold it against your bones knowing*
> *your own life depends on it;*
> *and, when the time comes to let it go,*
> *to let it go.*
>
> MARY OLIVER

INTERVENING IMPULSE: THE UNEXPECTED

Surrendering carries us further into moments of stillness, preparing the ground for the next phase of breaking open as we move closer to the turning point. Surrendering helps to create the space for intervening impulses to occur: sudden realizations, spontaneous insights, and sometimes alarming discoveries. A very common phenomenon observed in my research and validated by my personal experience is that, out of the depths and seemingly out of nowhere, we have a sudden wake-up call that opens our eyes when we least expect it.

Breaking open can be a moment of bottoming out, of feeling exposed, horrified, crazed, lost, finished, terrified. Just as easily, it can be a moment of revelation, an impulse toward the intuitive, the spiritual, toward a higher level of conscious awareness. The point is that it comes to us unbidden, catapulting us out of our previous way of viewing things, the mental attitude in which we were deeply embedded. It's as if the lights have been turned on and we can now see the very things that had eluded us before. Out of the blue, a whim, thought, comment, dream comes, and we feel the gridlock beginning to dissolve.

Here is how it feels on the inside, when *breaking open* happens:

- "I suddenly saw the complete denial. I was always thinking I could stop any time I wanted. I remember the moment I realized I could not go on like this one more day. It had to stop."
  Mike: Bottoming out after years of crippling addictive behavior

- "...a most amazing moment, as if all my priorities in life kind of reordered themselves, it came to me: I'd been living the wrong script. So many bad choices. I wasn't living my life according to what was most important to me and that I was going to do that regardless."
  Kim: Moment of clarity upon hearing the oncologist's report diagnosing cancer

- "I was in denial. One morning I woke up, and I knew that if I continued life as it was, I was going to get physically sick, that it could kill me. That was the morning that I started to be different."
  Jane: Abusive relationship, suddenly hitting the wall in terms of what she would tolerate

- "It was as if a signal came. I acted on the intuition, thank God, which was not my style. It's like I opened the one door that I had always kept completely closed."

Fran: Decision to adopt after years of miscarriages and multiple procedures that were painful and expensive, emotionally and physically

- "The thought came out of nowhere: DO NOT keep a journal of your disease. It's up to you to live with it. No joining MS support groups! No focusing on the issues surrounding it. NO, I just can't do it that way."
  Carol: Multiple sclerosis patient with sudden insight that made a massive difference in how she handled her illness

- "In the middle of a yoga class, with no expectation, I felt this for the first time in my life: I felt immersed in love, love and acceptance. It touched me very very deeply. I knew that whatever lies ahead can't be worse than where I've been."
  Lisa: In the middle of a painful divorce, an unexpected spiritual gift

- "I am not at all religious, but I felt guided like it came from my soul? Something was thawing out inside of me. Something was saying 'you need to trust, dare to trust.'"
  Ted: Radical change in career and lifestyle, the experience of relinquishing control of the situation

- "I suddenly realized! My stumps are exposed; I was exposed. It was total vulnerability and humiliation. Oh my God. People will see my body; they will look at me in horror, in disgust, will throw up. I had no protection! I hit bottom that day."
  Sarah: Survivor of auto accident, bottoming out through her worst nightmare of being seen as maimed

* "I could not accept that he was gone. I was basically in despair
  and waiting for nothing in particular. I had no real reason to go
  on without him, and then suddenly something opened up."
  Julie: Loss of spouse, finally surrendering to the reality of his
  death

* "It was a sudden realization: The marriage did not fail. It was a
  success. It's just that it was over, completed. It was time to go."
  Paul: Contemplating divorce after 30 years, permission came
  out of nowhere dissolving months of held anguish

* "For the first time in my life I felt that I knew who I was."
  Jonathan: During a silent meditation retreat, a discovery, a
  spontaneous inner awareness came out of the stillness

A STORY OF SURRENDER

There's a charming story of surrender that involves three frogs who fell
into a deep bucket of cream one night. The first frog was so overwhelmed
by what he saw as the hopelessness of the situation that he despaired
in fear and soon sank to the bottom. The second frog began frantically
leaping toward the rim; but without any leverage beneath him, he eventually exhausted himself and perished. The third frog was both realistic
and wise. He saw both the magnitude of the obstacles he faced and the
futility of leaping.

But he remained calm and considered a third option: to spend what
little time he had left doing what he did best, swimming the backstroke
while savoring the joyful exertion of the present moment. In the process
of doing just that, of enthusiastically surrendering, something unexpected happened: His paddling began to churn the cream into butter.
And to his amazement, he was soon able to easily leap out of the bucket
to solid ground. A very evolved frog!

David Whyte speaks to the experience of surrendering in an excerpt from his exquisite poem, *Sweet Darkness*:

> *The world was made to be free in*
> *Give up all other worlds*
> *except the one to which you truly belong*
> *Sometimes it takes the darkness and the sweet*
> *Confinement of your aloneness to learn:*
> *Anything or anyone*
> *That does not bring you alive*
> *Is too small for you.*

Just that one statement, "the world was made to be free in," is enough to knock open a door in one's mind. How free can anyone feel, tied up in knots of fear, anger, sadness, avoidance habits? In a way, all compulsive and addictive behaviors, including relatively benign ones like excess shopping, internet use, video games, TV, etc., serve the purpose of keeping change at bay. Indulging in them temporarily lowers our anxiety level, which is why they become our habit patterns.

But if we don't change, we don't grow. And if we don't grow, we're not really alive. Continuing our practice of stress-reduction skills is crucial at this point in order to become more adept at lowering our anxiety in a healthy and empowered way so that we can maintain progress. Without a reliable means of calming and steadying ourself, the current reality—the loss, the chaos, the uncertainty—can be just too overwhelming. Mindfulness and stress reduction do take some repeated effort initially, but they are profoundly liberating and empowering practices.

Taking deep cleansing in-breaths and slow full out-breaths on a very regular basis helps build the resilience we need to move forward through the process of breaking open. More and more, as we consciously surrender to what is, we will feel our sense of agitation lessening and our anxiety naturally decreasing. If our energy seems a little flat, that's okay; in fact, it's a good thing. Our vulnerability is at a record high during the breaking open phase, and there is a need for extra rest and support. Go with that.

Ideally, we are spending 15 to 20 minutes of every day practicing breathing mindfully, simply being here and now in the present moment, in a very safe, comfortable place where we can feel protected. Settle in. Sometimes it takes 10 minutes just for the sweet peaceful feeling of stillness to show up. But it can and will show up. We enhance the chances of that happening every time we set aside this quiet time. Healing time. Every time we practice this, it gets a little easier. Remember, we are grooving new neural pathways that will support us now and going forward.

Plus, it is from this place of inner peace, however fleeting, that our ability to act more constructively slowly begins to increase. A new sense of trust, a tiny hope begins to displace the recurring automatic negative thoughts that had preciously prevailed. This is also when we start to recognize that our meditation and relaxation practice has actually become a reliable new source of strength. Developing these strengths obviously takes some effort, but it's not as hard as going through life without them.

As our thinking becomes more objective, we begin to realize certain points that had eluded us earlier. Even though what's done is done, we can now see that we still have options. What threatens to hold us back at this point is fear of the unknown (what if things get even worse?), our inability to let go (then what?), and our deeply ingrained impulse to control the outcome. But we've become more and more aware of these very obstacles, and our confidence continues to grow as long as we practice staying open.

> *The soul should always stand ajar,*
> *ready to welcome the ecstatic experience.*
> EMILY DICKINSON

One of the surest signs of progress in the breaking open phase is our growing ability to tolerate nothingness. This is a feeling of emptiness, followed by a conscious surrender to whatever lies ahead. We move into that holy ground by asking more of the right questions. It is now important to identify how arresting thoughts, feelings, and images have stopped us from asking for what we really want (from life, from our relationships, from ourself). This is vital to understanding why we haven't asked these questions until now.

QUESTIONS FOR BREAKING OPEN

* Do you honestly feel you have a right to be happy?
* Do you really believe you have a right to live life in accordance with your truth?
* Are you disinclined to ask for something without a guarantee of results?
* Does your inner critic (inner tyrant) have the upper hand in your life, restricting your vision of what you know you need?
* Are you becoming more empowered in your ability to manage anxiety and tolerate uncertainty?

If *"resistance to tyranny is the secret of joy,"* as **Alice Walker** has suggested, how has your power and your joy in life been diminished by your inner tyrant? Now is the time to lift the veil and work with that. Ask yourself, take your time, and just see what rises to the surface. How have you boxed yourself in with premises that, though actually arbitrary, you have taken to be sacrosanct?

Staying trapped in a limited mind-set leads to stagnation, numbness, and depression. It leads to short-term self-negation and long-term destruction of one's potential. It leads to angst, despair, and inner violence—a subtle form of aggression toward oneself and sometimes toward others in the form of resentment. Sometimes we get stuck because we sense what we are looking for, but we don't want to risk going into unfamiliar territory to find it.

Ask courageous questions and watch what happens. Consider facing yourself and your biggest fear head on. No excuses. This takes courage, and yours has been steadily growing. If you feel exposed and vulnerable, like a crab that is shedding its too small shell, then you are on sacred ground. As Sufi Poet **Hafiz** says,

> *"The place where you are right now*
> *God circled on a map for you."*

EXERCISE: MORE QUESTIONS FOR BREAKING OPEN

* What painful unalterable reality have I avoided facing and accepting?
* What old belief/assumption do I need to let go of?
* Who or what is keeping me small?
* How have I been conspiring in my own diminishment?
* When will I release myself from this mind-trap?
* How can I make friends with uncertainty?
* What are the feelings and thoughts that stand in the way?
* What else can I let go of right now?
* What else ... ?

Letting go can mean many things. Sometimes it means forgiveness, not as an emotion, but as a very deliberate decision and as a spiritual gift to oneself—and not because the harm inflicted was so forgivable, but rather because holding onto anger only perpetuates and deepens the original damage. Letting go of the inexcusable is then a conscious choice that is essentially freeing and healing. It's no longer about the other person. It's about moving forward on our journey.

Forgiveness is about lightening our heart and spirit, unburdening our body and mind, so that we can be more fully alive. Letting go of anger brings a sense of inner spaciousness. It's also a way of breaking ground for new growth as opposed to trying to plant new seeds in hard-packed earth in need of aeration and motion. Like crocuses in the snow, half buried, but eagerly waiting to grow forth, we have a natural impulse for inner springtime. The practice of mindfully releasing, which is like melting the snow, applies to letting go of fear, sadness, lost beauty, past joys, and unfulfilled dreams as well. It's about allowing the weight of negative energy to dissolve. Most of our letting go is done in solitude, although it can often be a shared experience, facilitated by another's presence.

In addition to mindfulness, meditation, exploring, and surrendering, we need the support and comfort of at least one trusted ally who really understands what we are going through. It's crucial to make some healing connections in the form of a loyal friend, family member, therapist, counselor, or a new-found kindred spirit. Any relationship in which presence and authenticity is truly possible will support this process. A kind, focused, and respectful listener, who is genuinely there for us, conveying a sense of unconditional positive regard, can help us connect with and reveal what most needs to be expressed.

What is key is this: to be heard and witnessed for who we are and are not—and to be accepted and loved nonetheless. This is an important part of the opening process. It helps repair the brokenness, and we need one another for this to happen. Spending some time with an ally in this way is an important catalyst to healing and growing.

EXERCISE: AUTHENTIC ALLIES

- Who are your allies?
- Who can you really trust?
- Who can you count on to listen without judging you?
- Who has helped to liberate you to be yourself?
- Who says "come out" to you?
- With whom do you feel safe enough to say what must be said?

Growth demands a temporary surrender of security. Practicing surrender, even in a safe context in the presence of a close ally, is a brave and trusting act. Yet it is an integral part of the process of transformation, as revealed in this excerpt from **Marge Piercy's** poem, *The Magician*:

> *Give birth to me, sisters, in struggle we transform*
> *ourselves but how often, how often*
> *we need help to cut loose, to cry out, to breathe!*
> *This morning we must make each other strong*
> *Change is qualitative: we are*
> *each other's miracle.*

Regardless of the shape it takes or the depth of suffering that precedes it, surrendering is a powerful source of spiritual nourishment when we truly need it most. It is a prelude to our next new season of life, providing nourishment in our growth toward a higher level of conscious awareness. In the face of insurmountable adversity, we will either regress, or we will transcend. "When we are no longer able to change a situation, we are challenged to change ourselves," said **Viktor Frankl**, forever and for better.

This is the time to keep the file open inside ourselves and resist the tendency to reach premature conclusions, on either our own or others' lives. Just staying open is enough for now. A word of caution: Well-meaning others may express concern about your future, but they have blind spots too. Don't underestimate yourself and the great mystery that lies ahead of you, which may well include possibilities that neither you nor they could ever imagine.

EXPECT THE UNEXPECTED

When the Mt. St. Helens erupted in the 1980s, the volcano caused a 14-mile landslide, sterilizing 200 square miles of earth with pyroclastic flow. Scientific experts unanimously predicted that parades of pioneering species would lead the way and would alter the environment, making possible the second wave: First there would be lichen, then weeds and wildflowers, then herbs, then deciduous trees, then conifers, all rolling in from the edges. But when the experts gathered there 20 years later to track the progress, they discovered instead that most their predictions were completely inaccurate.

As it turned out, pockets of survivors (little biological legacies) had remained intact. Some were buried 600 feet deep in lava, and some rolled unscathed right along the top. This was a big epiphany for the scientists. Moles, gophers, ants, microbes, etc., had been deeply hidden and somehow spared, along with various seeds and saplings. Lupine seeds had blown in and found crevices for rooting. Rare and beautiful species that can create their own nitrogen began to flourish, unimpeded by more common plants that did not arrive until much later.

The reality that unfolded exceeded everyone's expectations. The point is, no one really knows what the future holds for you, including you. So why not surrender to the pure potentiality that really does exist in your life?

What lies behind us and what lies before us
are small matters next to what lies within us.
RALPH WALDO EMERSON

As we engage in this process of inner exploration and surrendering, penetrating illusions and uncovering aspects of our inner self and our outer situation, the need for self-acceptance and self-compassion becomes greater. It is when we are becoming emotionally naked to ourselves that we most need the warm blanket of self-compassion. This means inviting our inner critic to step aside and be silent.

"To a worm in horseradish, the whole world is horseradish," the old saying goes. But "You're braver than you believe, and stronger than you seem, and smarter than you think," said Christopher Robin to Pooh.

Now is the time to suspend self-judgment and be especially kind to ourselves. Fear brings contraction; joy brings expansiveness and energy.

Cultivating compassionate acceptance toward oneself is a kind of inner befriending process. It's about opening our heart in a new way, perhaps for the first time, as a shelter for all the disowned aspects of our being, parts that we have been ignoring for years without even realizing it. We are all suffering from some degree of self-aversion, often with very little conscious awareness of our unforgiving inner critic, the oppressive judge who is never quite satisfied with us as we are and never shuts up about it. It's about radical acceptance of those parts, about relating to them with gentleness, patience, understanding, and love, the way a loving and devoted parent would embrace a beloved and imperfect child. Practice giving safe refuge to the parts of yourself you'd rather not admit to. This is a time of surrendering and self-blessing.

Saint Francis and the Sow
The bud
stands for all things,
even for those things that don't flower,
for everything flowers, from within, of self-blessing;
though sometimes it is necessary
to reteach a thing its loveliness....
until it flowers again from within,
of self-blessing....
GALLWAY KINNELL

SUMMARY POINTS: CHAPTER 3:
BREAKING OPEN—SURRENDERING

"I really thought if something like this ever happened to me,
I would just die. But it all happened. And it didn't kill me"
EXCERPT FROM CASE STUDY

Cognition: Okay, what reality do I really need to accept? Examine deeply? Do differently? What do I need to let go of?

Premise: I have no idea what to do. I am lost. Nothing helps.

NATs softening: I give up. I surrender. I've hit bottom. Now what? [NATs diminish in intensity and begin to open to reasonable, realistic response (RRR).]

Emotions: Lessening of agitation; anxiety decreases, vulnerability increases: need for rest, support, protection

Physical: A softening: tension decreases; energy flat

Behavioral: Ability to act constructively slowly begins

Spiritual: Tiny hope, a new sense of trust; practice begins to be recognized as a source of strength.

Realization: Okay, what's done is done, but I still have options.

Catalysts and impediments:

Potential Pitfalls: fear of the unknown; impulse to control, inability to let go

Catalysts to growth: How can I find a way to make friends with uncertainty, with impermanence? How can I calm myself in the face of this new reality?

Practice: relaxation skills, mindfulness, meditation, openness to the unexpected

Exercise/Meditation: calm presence, letting go, self-compassion

The secret waits for eyes unclouded by longing

ZEN PROVERB

CHAPTER 4

Awakening—Breaking Through

This chapter tracks the fourth phase, awakening: breaking through the shell of our prior understanding and way of being.

As we enter the precarious territory where profound change is unfolding, our impulse to grow comes up against our tendency to regress. Inner resistance remains a persistent challenge during this emotionally fragile and unstable time. Key insights and spiritual skills help to keep us on track. There is a sense in the body as our perspective shifts into a higher level of conscious awareness.

"There is a felt sense that something has shifted, something's different, something unfamiliar and unexpected is happening. I have moments of feeling almost hopeful, for no particular reason."
EXCERPTED FROM CASE STUDY

TURNING POINTS

Buckminster Fuller was walking the beach one morning in a state of abject anguish and despair. Years before, he had succumbed to cultural and societal pressure, yielding, in his own words, to "fear, custom, and conditioning." He had suppressed his passion for invention and, instead, had agreed to work in the family business. Although he was doing a commendable job for the company, he also felt depleted and disconnected, initially from his dreams, then from his loved ones, and eventually even from himself. Trapped in a lifestyle that he found suffocating and grim, medicating himself with alcohol, Fuller got to the point where he saw no way out other than ending his life. He was seriously contemplating suicide on that blustery day as he walked along the beach, listening to the waves and watching the sky change colors.

He'd convinced himself that he and his family would be better off if he were dead and gone, rather than here and miserable. Just then, according to Fuller, a completely novel idea came to him out of the blue: What if **old Bucky** died—with his current obligations and restrictions intact—and a **new Bucky** got to live freely, with his own intuitive destiny as the blueprint? This question seemed like a totally outrageous notion at first, nothing more than another crazy, random thought. The compliant, miserable Bucky dead and buried and a newborn inventive, creative Bucky living joyfully in accordance with his true nature? A concept too preposterous to be taken seriously? Or a real option, too compelling to ignore?

As the afternoon unfolded, he became increasingly enthralled with the possibility of simply exercising his power to choose a radically different life. Somehow the shift began, and there he was on what became an unstoppable course, following what was for him the path of wholeness, on the most life-affirming and fulfilling journey he could ever have imagined. Fuller was profoundly changed in some ways and yet still the same in others. He remained devoted and loving to his wife and children. But he had experienced a major inner shift, a critical breakthrough in his path toward individuation and full autonomy.

He had released himself from the tyranny of being stuck in the life he was "supposed" to live, and freed himself to go forward and start living his dream. The rest is history, as they say. Fuller become one of the most respected innovators of his time—a renowned inventor, author, systems theorist, futurist, and designer of the geodesic dome and the biosphere. Had he stayed stuck within the confines of his early conditioning, he might have suffocated as a person, withered in the business world and/ or ended his life out of sheer hopelessness. Instead, he evolved. In his case, the breakthrough involved a classic ego-cide, as described in Chapter 3. His previous way of being had to actually die off to allow for a more autonomous and evolved way of being to be born.

Breaking through is the turning point phase of the transformative experience, the defining moment we've been moving toward right along. It is during this phase that an actual shift to a higher level of conscious awareness is experienced. It most often occurs once we have reached a point of utter surrender, a time of finally letting go and allowing ourselves to trust. Our previously held illusion—that we could ultimately control the situation (and alter reality) with our brains, our brawn, our intensity, and our Herculean effort—has proved to be untenable.

For those of us who do experience transformation, having watched our illusions unravel before us, we have found ourselves in a newfound place of terra firma—a place of mystery, light, and self-acceptance— with a budding sense that there is a larger reality into which we are now moving. We are on unfamiliar ground, on the one hand, and coming home to ourselves on the other. At first we are straddling both worlds, as captured in this poem by **Juan Ramon Jimenez.**

Oceans
I have a feeling that my boat
has struck, down there in the depths,
against a great thing.
And nothing happens!
Nothing ... Silence ... Waves ... Nothing happens
Or has everything happened,
and are we standing now, quietly, in the new life?

SHIFTS IN PERSPECTIVE

"Nothing happens, or has everything happened, and are we standing now, quietly, in the new life?" As we move into this phase, we are operating confidently now within the open space of a promising new premise: that we can and will find a way through this. Negative automatic thoughts that plagued us during the earlier stages are regularly being replaced with more rational realistic reappraisals of the situation. This in itself contributes to an empowered sense that we are stronger than this adversity, that we don't like it, but we can handle it. More and more, our new attitude is, *"I see myself moving forward; I know I can do this."*

Continued practice of mindfulness mediation and relaxation skills is steadily increasing our emotional and physical resilience. We are noticing that we have a greater ability to tolerate uncertainty and ambiguity, and this is a huge relief. Due to our supportive practices and to the process itself, our anxiety level is leveling out and normalizing during this phase. A sense of inner well-being is gradually restoring itself. Energy improves, along with better sleep patterns. The impulse to incorporate exercise and better nutrition into our life is often experienced again. We feel like we are really getting a grip.

Each of these factors combines and contributes to our increasing ability to self-regulate. From a behavioral standpoint, we have a greater ability to make conscious, deliberate choices. Spiritually, there is a gradual return of cautious optimism. We've been learning to become skillful at identifying and dealing with resistance by experiencing our familiar inner obstacles as workable now, rather than insurmountable. There is a growing sense that weight is lifting, angst dissolving, and energy shifting, along with a feeling of opening to new possibilities that we had not previously considered.

Self-reflection brings a renewed, overarching sense that this is our journey and that we are choosing to trust the process. We have increasing confidence, as deeper levels of self-awareness and self-loyalty become a more ingrained way of being. We now have the discipline of regularly asking ourselves—

* Going forward, what do I need more of?
* What do I need less of?
* What can I finally let go of now?
* What else?

The answers have opened our mind to where we need to go next. Exercises at the end of this chapter help to further ingrain a more courageous approach to life. We've developed a better understanding of where our personal pitfalls show up. If our progress seems to be halted, we are looking for root causes. Perhaps we've been yielding to fear, old and new, or to conditioning, the old habit patterns of the mind that no longer serve us.

Or maybe it's a flawed premise from the distant past that we need to recognize as merely a perceived limitation and potential inner obstacle, something to be transcended. These are the impediments to growth that we can keep working with effectively through mindfulness, self-observation, and awareness. This habit of opening to life brings an expansion of conscious awareness that is inherently liberating.

> *Every man takes the limits of his own vision*
> *for the limits of the world*
> ARTHUR SCHOPENHAUER

We can see more evidence of forward momentum as we face our adversity with strength and yet soften into it, as we consciously allow, rather than resist, the reality of the situation. There is an encouraging and disarming quality to this experience, as we cultivate acceptance of our current reality, including aspects that we previously believed were too impossible and unacceptable to tolerate. We are becoming more resilient.

Beauty blazes where eyes face truth fearlessly.

DAVID STEINDL-RAST

Our emotional stamina has been steadily increasing. We are expressing ourselves and standing up for ourselves in new and constructive ways. There is a lessening of the instinct to try and control what is beyond our control and an increase in coming to terms with uncertainty, letting go of attachment to outcome. It's about stepping into the mystery of our own life and knowing in our bones that, as **Mary Oliver** said in *The Journey*, you are "saving the only life you can save."

DEFINING MOMENTS

Reading the words of individuals in the midst of their turning point makes it possible to directly observe the transformation as it is happening. We can see their perspective shifting, dropping the old and birthing the new. The stories are uniquely personal—a divorce, an addiction, a diagnosis, a traumatic injury, or profound loss, etc., but a dynamic shift in perspective is universally experienced. Each of these people has a clear recognition that they are still struggling, but they are also very aware that something different is happening, something important is being discovered, and that they are proceeding, they are riding the wave of this new energy. What happens next are real turning points, the defining moments on their journey.

It is in the breaking through phase that we see the early stages of an actual shift into a higher conscious awareness. Most of the individuals quoted in the section that follows described the quality of their experience as being a moment of utter surrender to life, when they finally let go and began to trust. The illusion that they could control the situation with their reasoning powers and determination, working harder at old agendas, had already unraveled. They finally found themselves in a place of acceptance, often with a budding sense that there was a larger reality that they were moving into.

"There were many tests and further crisis, but I had hit that point you reach where you can't hold on anymore. That's when you have to surrender and say, okay, there's a greater plan, and I accept it. And then the transition began. I am not religious at all, but I felt supported by the universe, I really did. Whatever it takes, I can't betray myself anymore, I cannot, will not disregard my own (healthy) needs. It's time." TED

"It was like an epiphany. Everything shifted in a matter of seconds. And it came to me that there were only two things that were important to me: my relationship to my purpose in life (to God?) and my relationship to the people that I really loved. Nothing else was really that important. I was in a very centered place." KIM

"I had been pretending for so long, hiding out in denial, and I suddenly came to a still point. It was like an intuitive message that I had to be more of a witness. I had to be able to listen differently. I had to really look at what was happening in my marriage. It was right there in front of me all along, but I guess I wasn't ready to see it. That's when I began to see my life for what it was. No more illusions." JANE

"I was sitting there trapped and exposed, in total despair, when it came like a bolt to me: Just live your life, live how you do it. Just do it, and don't pay any attention to how they look at you. You could be destroyed by that. That was my first real awakening of dealing with being 'in the chair.'" SARAH

"Those words, 'Who knows what wars are going on where the spirit meets the bone?' really hit me in a deeply personal way. It was a meltdown, in a good way, something thawing out inside, and I started to feel compassion and empathy toward myself, real appreciation of myself, my courage, my humanity, instead of seeing myself as a failure. That was the beginning of the change." FRAN

"I started realizing I had been teaching one thing and living something else, for years and years. I knew that I finally had to be authentic. Spirituality, meditation, yoga—they had helped me move into the fear and move through it. Now the shift was finally happening in my life. It was a feeling of integrity that I hadn't ever had before." LISA

"And then this little woman, this total stranger, came over to me at the end of the AA meeting, and she said, "Do you want to live or do you want to die?" And I just sat there. I couldn't speak. And then she said, "God loves you; he's got plans for you." And that's when everything started to turn for me. It was the beginning of acknowledging something greater— even if only mythology, still—and being part of that in some way. These people care about me. My life can have meaning. I can heal, and I can help others heal." MIKE

"The basic question I had not focused on was, 'Who am I besides his ex-wife?' All my attention was on him and his cruel behavior. I suddenly saw it: All the agonizing in the world was not helping me one single bit, it was only hurting me, holding me back. He was unaffected by my anger and pain, oblivious. So what's the point? I decided then and there that I had to choose. I had to work on my own garden, or I would wither as a person. It was horrifying to think about, but it made a big difference." LAURA

"I was walking the beach, watching the waves roll in, when it came to me, the realization that I would have to just risk all and completely trust, that whatever difficult consequences were inevitable, I could accept them. I would be able to handle it, whatever it was. It's all a matter of trust."
PAUL

"I went just for a rest, to be quiet and recover myself, but I had a spiritual change there. I realized that I had no sense of self-love before. I finally learned how to cry. Major grief came out, free grief, like orgasm really. It takes over the whole body. I could never have done this earlier on."
ALISON

"It came to me out of nowhere, this stark realization: There's nothing wrong with me. I just don't fit the culture! That was when I realized I had an intuitive self that I could rely on for guidance, and that was when I began to see myself as okay, as valuable really, and even mythic in a way. And I felt peaceful for no reason." PETER

"It was out of the blue. I just suddenly saw that I had a choice in this. And I made the decision right then and there that I would make it (the disease) the smallest possible part of my life. This was such a huge relief to me. It was the turning point." CAROL

"At an Alanon meeting, I heard them say, 'Recover or repeat; recover or repeat.' It ripped into me in a powerful way. I realized I can't live this way. I had to change myself. I had to drop the rage, let the anger go. It saved my life. I actually started meditating, me the cynic! I saw how badly I needed love and support too, needed healing, and I was learning to open to it, to accept it from these people. That's when I saw what years of loneliness had been doing to me." DONNA

"I can't explain it really. I just suddenly felt totally and completely surrounded by love, just filled with love. I went from feeling devastatingly horrible to feeling filled and surrounded by love, and I knew I was going to be okay. Is that what grace is? I don't know." ANNE

"There is a felt sense that something has shifted, something's different, something unfamiliar and unexpected is happening, I have moments of feeling almost hopeful again, for the first time in so long, and for no particular reason. 'I can do this,' is my first thought now. I'll be okay." BRAD

"I suddenly recognized, and then felt convinced, that my life wasn't over. As a physician, I had the means and the right to end it now, but I decided to choose life. I suddenly had a sense of unfinished business, a feeling that there was something important and mysterious that still could happen. I still have something to learn, to give, to contribute. I'm a staunch atheist and a scientist, but I began practicing a little meditation every day. I was amazed to feel oddly peaceful, even happy, in the present moment, even though I still considered myself to be quite depressed, technically." JULIE

"I'd been reading Proust, Remembrance of Things Past, and somehow it just came to me. I just got that we are only ever living in the present, and everything we call the past is happening in the present. It's right here in this moment, as a thought or as an image, and it was a remarkable shift." JONATHAN

The intellect has little to do on the road to discovery....
In the middle of difficulty lies opportunity.
There comes a leap in consciousness, call it intuition or what you will,
and the solution comes to you, and you don't know how or why.
ALBERT EINSTEIN

SIX STORIES

Although the people quoted earlier reveal the commonality in their experience, the details surrounding each turning point couldn't be more dissimilar. There isn't a single representative narrative. But the following stories are six dramatic examples of how the breaking through phase can unfold.

DANIELE: *"I actually felt joyful for the first time in over a year."* Daniele had already spent a full year recovering from the trauma of being raped by a friend of the family at the age of 17. Although many things had been very helpful that year, particularly her parents' love, a supportive therapist, and immersion in her academics, Daniele still remained socially withdrawn, plagued with a sense that she was irreparably damaged and broken. Like most victims of sexual abuse, she continued to feel both violated and guilty at the same time. Though obviously innocent, she had become immobilized by shame, never wanting anyone to find out what had happened to her.

She had also become more and more isolated, as if somehow needing to repent for this crime committed against her. Hiding out whenever possible, she felt energetically lifeless and depressed, totally disconnected from her sexuality, and fearful of being around people in general, especially men.

She had more or less maladapted to the idea of living a very sheltered and limited existence for the rest of her life. She had no vision of where to go from here—until the day that she experienced her turning point when she least expected it: her amazing breakthrough.

Slumped over a calculus book, Adrianna was studying algorithms one evening when her college roommate came back to the dorm with an Electric Gypsyland CD. Then she turned up the volume and started belly dancing around their room. However foreign, the sound and rhythm were so irresistible to Daniele that she was on her feet in a nanosecond, moving in synch with the music, swirling her body with a surprising lack of inhibition. Although she had never belly danced before, Daniele was clearly a natural at it. She began dancing with abandon and self-expression as if she'd been studying it for years.

Thirty minutes later, Daniele was drenched with sweat and beaming with joy. Something profound had just begun to happen. She felt instinctively that she was no longer disconnected from her body. She had come home to herself. The intensity and spontaneity of this full body exertion seemed to heal the split between her mind and her body in a way that nothing else had touched. That was the day Daniele came back to life, in a very new way on her journey toward wholeness.

It felt amazing to actually be "in her body," joyfully present again for the first time in over a year. Belly dancing for a while, almost every day, became part of Daniele's healing and part of her new life. The healing process took a little time, proceeding degree by degree. First movement, then joy, then sensuality, then a feeling of wholeness returned. And in a matter of days she began inching out of her self-imposed exile and was able to handle being with her close friends and participating in small gatherings again.

Two years later, Daniele was leading social action groups on campus and becoming a student activist on human rights, raising awareness for victims of oppression, such as the migrant farm workers in her region. The most triumphant moment so far in her healing journey involved being a keynote speaker at an intercollegiate rally, addressing women's safety issues and the growing problem of date rape on college campuses.

On that occasion, she amazed herself by acknowledging before a crowd for the very first time that she herself was a survivor of rape. Her courage in speaking out was met with great respect and awe and likely contributed to the healing of other survivors who were no doubt present. Today, Daniele is a beautiful inspiration to everyone who meets her, a true spiritual warrior in the best sense of that term: brave, compassionate, empowered, kind, authentic, joyful, and whole.

JANE: *"An unhappy ending was better than unending unhappiness."* It took many years for Jane, age 46, to reach her turning point, (see page 15); but once she summoned the courage to surrender, she was able to really witness what was going on in her marriage and confront the underlying issues, the ones she had instinctively avoided facing for many years. Once that phase began, she knew there was no turning back. Various personal traits had been conspiring to keep her small enough to stay in what amounted to emotional captivity.

Prepared to be self-sacrificing for the greater good, Jane was not a quitter. The whole idea of a getting a divorce represented failure to her. Then there was the anticipated guilt of being the one who would be initiating it. Ironically, despite the fact that she had been the target of her husband's emotional abuse for years, she hated the thought of hurting him.

Reading endless relationship books on staying versus leaving had kept her at an impasse. Reaching the solution was simply not available through making checklists of pros and cons. All the cognitive and analytical skills in the world were only increasing her frustration without moving her toward a decision. Nor did it help to agonize about her feeling of being trapped and her worse fear of remaining trapped.

Years of being maneuvered and manipulated had left her with a huge case of self-doubt. Could really she justify ending the marriage? Was she overestimating the negatives? Even if she wasn't, did she still have the ability to make it on her own? Maybe; maybe not. "If I leave, who will I be besides his ex-wife? Pathetic," she thought. Her self-esteem had been eroded to the point where her self-confidence was woefully diminished.

Second-guessing herself became a way of life. Would her family and friends understand and really get it? Or would they side with him? He had, after all, the ability to be charming, persuasive, engaging, and endearing when he wanted to be. So there she was, disabled by emotional abuse, disempowered by fear, wallowing in despair and self-aversion at her own ineptitude.

Jane had lost her ability to be even decisive, let alone take any courageous action. She had been cycling this way for years when something started shifting. It was during a series of yoga classes that her turning point occurred. Jane had signed up just to relieve some tension, lower her anxiety, relax her body, and maybe tone it up a bit. She expected nothing more.

Her yoga teacher's invitation to suspend thinking and try letting go of the past and the future while focusing on breathing in and breathing out through every posture, seemed preposterous. For one whole hour? This sounded like a rather indulgent idea, kind of naïve, and wildly impractical, to Jane. The only reason she was ready to give it a chance was that she was at the end of her rope.

So she gradually allowed herself to trust in the idea of cultivating surrender as part of spiritual practice. She kept hearing that it wasn't all about exertion, but rather about mindfulness, about the balance of effort and ease, discipline and surrender. At first these ideas were nothing more than foreign concepts to her, surely not a practical strategy for finding solutions in life.

But she found herself opening to the possibility that to surrender on some level could be a conscious choice in service of growth. It was not easy to take a chance on what can be described as a trans-rational approach, temporarily suspending ordinary reasoning powers in order to go beyond them. She had been educated to see the human mind as primary.

But she allowed herself to trust, to shift out of problem-solving mode, if only during yoga class, for a 60-minute experiment each week. And that experience in turn planted a seed for change inside of her. Jane sensed it instinctively: that if she could do this in yoga class, she could do it in life.

In time, the yogic practice of being in her body, as opposed to staying lost in her head, added yet another dimension that supported Jane's healing and growth. Change was happening, on a very subtle but palpable level. She was coming into her own. She was ripening. It was one evening, coming out of resting in savasana pose, deeply absorbed in the present moment, that Jane had the actual experience of breaking through.

A profound insight from the unforgettable Mary Oliver poem came to her unbidden in that very moment: This is your "one wild and precious life." Right then, Jane knew that she needed to risk speaking her truth and that one unhappy ending was better than unending unhappiness—that getting a divorce, frightening as it seemed, was better than staying trapped in an abusive marriage. For Jane, it came down to a matter of self-loyalty, and it was long overdue. She still had many rough hurdles and harrowing challenges ahead, but she kept hearing the phrase, "my soul knows it's safe," which came to her from who knows where?

DAN: *"But wait, my life matters too."* No one was more disillusioned than Dan to see how his promising life had unfolded. He had always been a natural leader—admired, responsible, respected, and loved, even as a very young man. Sincere, kind, accomplished and bright, he excelled in his profession as well as his family life. But although Dan's life looked wonderful from the outside, deep down there was a void and a sadness. Like Ted in a sense, he was too functional for his own good.

Having no stomach for conflict, Dan strove to maintain harmony and fill in the gaps wherever possible. But in doing so he had put everyone else's needs–his wife's, his two daughters', his employer's—above his own, eventually to his serious detriment. Somehow he always seemed to lack the time and the energy to pursue his creative gifts and interests. There was no space available for friendships or athletics in his demanding schedule. Dan's life had become way out of balance with his obligations to others taking up seven days a week.

Years of putting his own needs last had evidently begun to take their toll. The only respite he was allowing himself was found in smoking marijuana. Although Dan had dabbled casually in drugs in college, that context was recreational. He certainly never considered himself an addict ever in his life. He was convinced that he could give up smoking pot any time he wanted to stop.

As an outlet from all the pressures at work and at home, it was easy enough to rationalize it, mainly to himself. He needed to take the edge off now and then, sometimes weekly, sometimes daily. And smoking pot hadn't caused him any real problems that he was aware of. He'd never missed a day of work, clear evidence there was no problem, in his mind. But age 49, he had a major wake-up call, which started subtly and became a life-altering recognition of what was missing. It was an intuitive opening that led to change and growth.

Approaching his 50th birthday turned out to be a pivotal period for Dan, call it grace or serendipity or whatever you like. There was no big drama to his breakthrough. For Dan, after decades of denial and defensiveness, it was a moment of authentic self-confrontation, followed by a surrender to reality that brought about a major shift in his perspective. Commuting home from work on the train, he had just been reading his annual peer review, where his many competencies were recognized and his areas of growth were named. It was all familiar stuff and it was all good, as usual. He felt recognized and gratified, justifiably. But it was then that the question hit him like a bolt: "If someone did an honest review of your inner life, how would that look? You're almost 50. What are you becoming? Where are you headed?"

He was stunned to see the contrast in his private life—between his external competencies (pride in being an excellent provider, husband, and father) and his internal ones, his areas of personal growth (a gaping void). After years of denial and resistance to facing this, he simply dropped his defenses and allowed himself to take a closer look at who he was deep inside.

That was the moment when Dan began to see his life with new eyes. Feeling deep sadness, tinged with shame, he dared to actually look into that void for the first time. Previously he was either too depleted from taking care of others' needs to actually examine his own, or he was too zoned out in stony exhaustion. Or he was recovering from zoning out. He had already wasted days, nights, years of his potential, basically lost in space. How had he not noticed?

In Dan's case, it wasn't that he was doing too much of the wrong thing, although smoking pot obviously has its hazards. It was more that Dan wasn't doing enough of the right thing for who he was, who he had the potential to be. He'd once been a terrific athlete, had creative interests, lots of good friends, a fabulous sense of humor, and tons of energy for life. How had his once full life narrowed down like this? When did it happen? Where did it all go?

"Up in smoke" was the intuitive answer that came to him like a bolt from nowhere. The more he inquired within, the clearer it became. The contrast between who he'd once been and how he was living was just too alarming to ignore. That was the day he began to change, to heal what needed to be healed and to grow into who he had the innate capacity to be.

Dan's first efforts to turn his life around were hard work, and he did most of it alone with only occasional visits to a life coach. The toughest challenge involved making the initial commitment to be accountable to himself for various goals, the first of which involved weaning himself from marijuana. Until he redefined pot as a serious obstacle to his potential for joy and for life, that commitment simply was not going to happen.

For all his confidence in most areas, Dan was actually fearful, after all these years, of giving up smoking pot, fearful that he might not be able to decompress or lighten up or go to sleep without it. At the very least, he would have to admit he had a dependency, which was not easy for Dan to do. Next, he would have to learn some stress-reduction techniques so that he could lower his anxiety in a reliable way. Learning to release tension through body scanning and focused breathing was the first step.

Once he discovered some free apps and great sources for accessing downloadable material, he was well on his way to naturally regulating his stress level. It was very empowering. He then became more skillful at creatively visioning his ideal self and applied creative visualization methods quite effectively. And then came the work of developing new interests, plus cultivating old and new friendships that were supportive, fun, healing connections for him. Obviously this did not happen overnight. But at least he was now on track.

There were multiple challenges for Dan, but in time he met each of them head on. The biggest hurdle for him by far was the first: getting past self-deception and denial. Witnessing the connection between his thoughts, his emotions, and his habitual behaviors became his new growth area. Developing strategies to stay on track followed.

Being able to trust the process greatly enhanced his steady progress in moving forward. Feeling increasingly alive, his confidence grew with each new conscious step on the path. "Whatever lies ahead, I know now that I can and will deal with it." This positive statement became one of his guiding affirmations, along with the insight, "But wait, my life matters too," which became his handrail to the life that was waiting for him.

It took time, and he sometimes drew criticism from his family for being less available. After all, it had been very convenient to have him working overtime for them all those years. But in the end, this change led his family members to become more self-sufficient, which was healthier for everyone in the end. Looking back from where he is today, amazed at his own journey, Dan is vibrantly healthy, physically and emotionally, and more creative, happy, exuberant, and energized than he has felt in years. He embraced his crisis as opportunity. He has reclaimed his autonomy, his power, and his life.

KIM: *"All my priorities shifted in that moment."* She was 51 years old and in seemingly perfect health, but a series MRIs and biopsies confirmed the diagnoses that Kim had stage three breast cancer. After the initial experience of disbelief, fear, and anger, she collapsed into a state of grief.

She didn't want to die, she didn't deserve to die, and she just could not believe it was happening to her of all people. She was in fact self-righteous about exercising regularly, eating fairly well, and not having smoked in thirty years. Kim felt betrayed by fate, betrayed by the system, and even betrayed by her own body. Her tension level was so elevated, she felt as if she were gasping for air half the time.

She had been advised to practice diaphragmatic breathing, and as a nurse she understood the clinical benefits of doing this. But she could barely make the effort. About all that she could muster was to practice a little mindfulness from time to time.

She had been attempting to do this, trying to be in the here and now, wanting to let go of past and future, trying to trust, although it all seemed too strange and simplistic to be taken seriously. Yet practicing mindfulness actually afforded her a few random moments of inner peace when her mind would finally quiet down, if only to flare up again minutes later.

One morning, in the midst of an overwhelming sadness and despair in which she felt tightly gripped, her turning point came out of the blue. It began with a sense that her armor was letting down and a feeling of lightness flowing was into her. She was standing in her kitchen, mindfully absorbed in the present moment, slicing apples. What followed was a wave of humility, a massive attitude adjustment, and then a spontaneous reordering her priorities.

Kim was still in her kitchen, but she was standing in a different world. She suddenly saw how hard she had been on everyone. She saw the unrealistic demands she had placed on herself to keep up a good front with others and how painfully her ego had been getting in the way. She saw her rigid expectations that she should always be in control and somehow be superior at all times, which was clearly unsustainable right now. She saw both the hard-heartedness and self-aversion that had fueled this behavior for so long. And she began to thaw out, in a good way.

Until then was she truly unaware of just how condescending and dismissive she had been, how impatient and hypercritical with her staff at the hospital and with her husband and children at home. In that moment of clarity, she also saw how self-serving and superficial she had been in her relationships across the board. For Kim, her breakthrough involved a massive change of heart. However long she'd be able to survive, she was determined to live her life with real gratitude and appreciation for those with whom she came in contact on a day-to-day basis.

Above all, she sensed this with a wave of humility, a very new experience for Kim. Out of character, she joined a circle of survivors and began sharing respectfully with people whom she had previously regarded as beneath her. She began living her life differently, as if every moment and every person mattered. It took a terminal diagnosis for her to snap out of her self-absorbed superiority, but in her case, she actually says she is grateful to have had a second chance to live a more conscious and compassionate life for as long as it does last.

SARAH: *"I can't let them matter, or I'm their prisoner for life."* Sarah's story is so rare that you might question my decision to include it here at all. However its message is also so universal that I feel it really must be told. It's about being trapped in suffering, then surrendering to reality, transcending fear, and experiencing the sweetness and power of emotional freedom. You may remember from the first chapter that Sarah lost both legs in an automobile accident when she was 35 years old.

Between her high tech wheel chair, precision devices, and handicap-designed car, she had become a wiz at managing the activities of daily living at home. But in her inner life, Sarah remained deeply and increasingly troubled. "The most depressing part for me was the way people look at you. I was always so terrified of embarrassment, about facing people, always hiding my body. I was so miserable, so alone." At 35, she was well on her way to becoming a recluse. When she did venture out with her wheelchair, she always took elaborate steps to cover her stumps with long pants and heavy throws.

The thought of being seen as disfigured had been terrifying to her until one hot summer day when Sarah broke through the very fear that had been so emotionally disabling. She'd been wearing shorts at home and had dashed out of her apartment in her wheelchair to pick up a last-minute recipe ingredient at a local grocer.

When she suddenly realized, there in the market, that her stumps were completely uncovered and exposed, Sarah was immobilized with the thought, "Oh my God, people will see my body, they will look at me in disgust, maybe throw up." It was a paralyzing moment of humiliation, horror, vulnerability, and abject fear. Sarah described it as feeling intensely aware, totally trapped, and completely defenseless. "I hit bottom that day." Yet deep inside of her, an illusion that she had fought so hard to keep up had started collapsing, in a good way, and she went with it. Her anguish began to spontaneously dissolve.

From the rubble of that momentary surrender came a priceless gift that was nothing short of a crucial transformative opening, an experience of liberation. In her own words: "That's when the shift happened, right in the middle of my worst fear, I suddenly said to myself: "I can't let them matter, or I'm their prisoner for life. Just don't give a damn. As long as you keep your focus on worrying that people are going to stare at you, you can't really live. No! Don't buy that. You can do anything you want. You can wear shorts! But just don't pay attention to what's out there. Just live your life. Live how you do it. Just do it and don't pay any attention to how they see you. You could be destroyed by that.

"And that was my first real awakening of dealing with being in the chair. You know you could get to the point where you can't go anywhere. It would be so stifling. You have to come to grips with that. Get beyond that. Be yourself. It was just my own insecurity. But I can't get caught up in that. People may be cruel sometimes, but you can't let that stop you."

To this day, Sarah is an inspiration to everyone who meets her or even sees her from a distance. Aside from her community of students and friends, total strangers have come up to her on the street and in various public places, just to tell her how much they admire her courage and her style. She moves around with such great energy and joi de vivre, you would think she had not a care in the world. Here is a woman who, despite a massive physical handicap, has a black belt in positive attitude—fun-loving, vivacious, emotionally generous, and living, breathing proof that we can transcend limitations and totally enjoy being all that we still can be, no matter what.

BRENDA: *A memoir moment.* There have actually been many significant turning points in my life so far, but one that I will relate here happened on the first Thanksgiving after ending my 28-year marriage. Having made it through the multilevel ordeal and upheaval of divorce, I was so looking forward to sharing Thanksgiving in my cozy new quarters with my three grown children, each recently out of college. It was beyond strange to be solo after being married most of my life, and I wanted to create a sense of continuity, of family and home life for my children despite all the changes. Months were spent busily preparing our home for their visit. But as it turned out, each of my children was obligated with their brand new jobs on the other side of the country, and none could travel home that year.

Of course, I was very proud of them for being responsible about their newly landed jobs and for living their young lives as independent adults now. At the same time, it was secretly really tough to be entirely alone on what had been a meaningful family holiday for all of my previous life. At first I was overwhelmed with a sense of grieving, feeling broken and lost.

But as with all crises, it was also an opportunity to grow. It involved facing and letting go of my attachment to the past, to being part of the family and to mothering—at least in the way that I had been for so many years. Where could I go? Where did I belong now? Who was I, in this new context? It was not until I fully opened to the pain, expressed it freely, and surrendered to the deep feelings of sorrow and loss that I finally reached a still point from which my turning point emerged.

It was then that the impulse came to me out of the blue: Why not spend Thanksgiving Day at a hospice residence, with whoever is there, total strangers, for their last Thanksgiving? Since I had previously worked as a volunteer in my local hospice program, I assumed that my offer to help on Thanksgiving would be accepted without question. However, when I called the residence in another town, offering to volunteer for the day, the head nurse said absolutely not.

Because I had not been through their specific training program, I would not be permitted there. Somehow her rejection seemed too sense-less to be the final word. So I then called the reception desk and asked when visiting hours were on Thanksgiving. The answer? "All day, for family and friends."

On Thanksgiving morning, off I went, dressed for this very special occasion. Pausing at the reception desk, I carefully signed my name in the guest book as simply "Friend of the Family." No doubt, this act seemed inconsequential to the receptionist, but for me, it was an intense and deeply significant turning point. I may not have had a husband now or had my beloved children within reach, but I was still part of a family, the human family, and I was determined to give myself wholeheartedly to it for now.

I spent most of the day with patient after patient, just being present with them in the moment, sometimes silently. But once I entered David's room, I knew it was where I should stay. The entire evening was spent with this fragile, pale, beautiful 35-year-old patient, 5 feet-11 inches and barely 100 pounds with just a few weeks to live. We talked, he slept, and he woke again. That evening, I fed him what was to be his last Thanksgiving dinner: some spoonfuls of jello with melon cubes, which was all he could swallow anymore.

He whispered, and I listened to stories of his happy childhood in Jackson, Mississippi, his sweet and beloved grandma, his joys, his loves, his favorite flavors, now just sensory memories: a good cup of coffee and a piece of pie. We laughed together and cried together. He asked me if I was his angel. "No, just your friend,"

I said. Yes, "Friend of the Family."

It was one of the most intensely memorable Thanksgivings ever. Life-changing, really. All day long, I knew something in me was dying, and something else was being born. "Nothing happens or has everything happened, and are we standing now, quietly, in the new life?" as Jimenez had said. I tucked David in for the night and drove home, stunned with gratitude.

TREASURE IN RUIN

These are a few of the stories, each of which illustrates in its own way how it feels to experience a major inner shift. We've seen how these individuals spontaneously experienced a meaningful change right in the midst of their chaos, fear, and despair. For the first time, these men and women were actually able to surrender, to move through fear, to risk uncertainty, to release their grief, to believe in themselves, to let go of their terror, to let go of anger, to gain a sense of acceptance, to pray for help, to feel supported by the universe or by God, to open to community, to make the decision to change—in short, to trust the process of life on a whole new level.

They described this as a profoundly new awareness and higher consciousness in which their perception of themselves and their relationship to their loved ones, to the world, to their purpose in life, sometimes to God or the great mystery, and even to life itself, underwent a dramatic and radical shift. In almost every case, this turning point occurred only after a period of intense turmoil and pain in which these individuals felt they were absolutely up against a wall. And then the opening came to them.

*There is always treasure in ruin. Why do we not
seek the face of God in the devastated heart?*

RUMI

Even when the shift occurred in a seemingly sudden way, as an unanticipated burst of awareness, it was really more of a phoenix rising from the rubble. It could also be described as a surpassing experience in which the individuals moved beyond their previous identity to include a wider and deeper perspective with regard to themselves, their adversity, and their life. Most often, they didn't see it coming. But they invariably described it as being liberating in a profound and powerful way.

Despite the dissimilarity in outer forms and details, each of these people experienced their breakthrough only at the very desperate point of total recognition that the crisis they were facing was beyond their personal control. They suddenly got it that they simply could no longer continue in their preexisting mind-set or consciousness. What was happening was huge enough to actually be a threat to their life, either because the suffering had finally become so intense and chronic that they could no longer tolerate it or because they literally knew they could very easily die, unless something changed within themselves, which is key.

*When we are no longer able to change a situation,
we are challenged to change ourselves.*

VIKTOR FRANKL

Until that point, their focus had been on rearranging their outer circumstances, like the deck chairs on the Titanic, in an attempt to control or at least manipulate the external conditions of their lives. They were assuming that, if they could just get the pieces right, have it the way they wanted it, their life would work, it would somehow make sense. This was the general illusion, regardless of the duration or of the details.

It's interesting to note that many of these people did have insights before, sometimes for years, either about the importance of the inner world or even about their need for transcendence, but until they reached the proverbial wall—the outer limits of their previous way of relating to things—and then actually surrendered, they remained very painfully in place, trapped in their old attitudes and illusions.

> *Ruin or recovery ... are from within.*
> EPICTETUS

They may have been diligently trying different strategies to comfort or placate or improve themselves. They all had made some minor changes here and there. But they were still relating to themselves and life as though it were entirely up to them alone—as if the burden were on their shoulders to get it right, to make the right decision, to take the right course of action, to find the right whatever. And all the while fearing that they might not have what it takes to do it anyway. They might not be that lucky. They might have to live small and die small.

All that their futile efforts had brought them was the illusion of progress and then further pain and entrenched fear, which in turn was followed by intensified efforts or despair. This is the wheel of samsara described in Buddhist psychology, the endless frustration and suffering that keeps cycling until we penetrate the illusion of the ego and free ourselves from the unconscious limitations of the unawakened existence.

> *The important thing is this:*
> *to be able at any moment to sacrifice*
> *what you are for what you could become.*
> CHARLES DU BOIS

When the turning point actually occurred, it was not so much a matter of cognitive choice as it was a sudden awareness—an experience of the sheer impossibility of living otherwise. It's as if there was a moment of awakening, a spiritual impulse, a grace in which they sensed the sea change and gave themselves over to it as their smaller identity began to dissolve. This relates to what Dr. Rosen called ego-cide, as described earlier. Finally they began to recognize and accept that they alone could not control the outcome, and they had to now surrender to something indefinable, to the mystery, to a higher power, a caring universe, an archetypal self, a benevolent God—to whatever concept allowed them and enabled them to let go and to trust and to transcend from where they had been.

Evolution is self-realization through self-transcendence.
ERICH JANSTCH

This shift was more than another mental construct in their heads. It registered in their physical, emotional, and spiritual being. By many reports, there was a spontaneous openness to the idea of soul or spirit operating in their life and with it a sense of faith that they would make it. Some felt that they were part of something larger than the ordinary realm of consciousness and that they were somehow mysteriously protected. They still had to do the work, so to speak, but it no longer seemed like an entirely solo mission. And this really made a difference.

Dramatic and lasting change for the better springs in part from radically shifting your perspective of who you are and what your true options are. This most essential change, the one from which all other changes arise, is a shift in how you view the world and your place in it. As our perception broadens, a whole array of unconsidered possibilities becomes available for us to explore, increasing our opportunities for consciously choosing how we want to be in this precious life.

You don't get to choose how you're going to die, or when.
You can only decide how you're going to live. Now.

JOAN BAEZ

Many believed that their journey had taken on a somewhat heroic quality as a result of their expanded awareness. We are all wired for exactly this kind of change and growth. We are immensely capable of learning and becoming adept at stress-reduction skills and at cognitive reframing skills, replacing negative automatic thoughts with more realistic appraisals, to naturally lower our anxiety level, increasing our confidence that we can handle whatever is ahead.

These skills naturally develop greater emotional resilience in us, an ability to ride the waves of uncertainty and ambiguity with abiding calm. Our emotional stamina increases as body awareness, deep breathing, and mindfulness practice contribute to our having better energy, better sleep patterns, and an enhanced sense of well-being. From a spiritual and emotional standpoint, this when we notice a gradual return of cautious optimism. Weight is lifting, dissolving, and shifting. We are opening up to new considerations that previously had eluded us. We are breaking through to the next phase.

RESISTANCE

Exhilarating and miraculous as it all is, the experience of breaking through is not the end point of the process or even of this phase. It is inevitable that we will eventually, sooner rather than later, encounter some form of resistance that threatens to halt our progress. To stay on track, anticipation is key so that we can handle the resistance with awareness, mindfully and skillfully. This involves building on skills that we've been developing right along. The potential pitfall at this point involves the pull of the past on us, the momentum of old ways, our conditioning, the habit patterns of the mind, our behavioral tendencies, and the flawed premises that inform the outmoded tapes still playing in our heads now and again. Unfortunately, resistance seems so be part of our DNA as well.

STAYING TRAPPED, *INSTINCTIVELY*

One night I baited a Havahart® trap in hopes of capturing and relocating a feral cat that had been terrorizing my very elderly house cat each night for weeks. When the trap slammed shut in the middle of that night, we could all hear the raging sounds of a trapped animal screeching and pouncing against the cage door, trying to free itself. I assumed that the mission was accomplished. What I found instead the next morning was not the feral cat I'd expected to see, but a young raccoon sleeping peacefully in the trap.

After protesting wildly hours before, he eventually quieted down and had drawn pine needles into the cage, creating a plump round mattress for himself, and settling in for a good night's sleep. The next morning, the raccoon watched closely as I carefully opened the trap door and stepped away so that he could have a clear exit.

But did he budge? Not an inch. The very trap that he had railed against hours earlier was now his comfort zone, his new cage of choice. Although nothing stood in the way of his claiming his freedom, he chose captivity in that moment. We all do at times. This book is about encountering the trap doors inside ourselves and growing the courage to open them.

When we no longer know what to do
we have come to our real work and
when we no longer know which way to go
we have begun our real journey.
The mind that is not baffled is not employed.
The impeded stream is the one that sings.
WENDELL BERRY

*"There is a felt sense that something has shifted, something's different,
something unfamiliar and good is happening. I feel hopeful."*
EXCERPT FROM CASE STUDY

Cognition: I am struggling, but something's happening, being discovered, and I am proceeding. Going forward I will need more _____ and less of _____. What else do I need to let go of? What else?

Premise: I can and will find a way through this.

NAT moves toward RRR: I don't like it but I can handle it. I am stronger than this problem.

Emotions: increased resilience and, as a consequence, greater ability to tolerate uncertainty and ambiguity

Physical: anxiety level normalizes; a sense of well-being begins to be restored; energy improves with better sleep, nutrition, exercise

Behavioral: increased ability to make conscious choices; learning to deal more skillfully with resistance

Spiritual: gradual return of cautious optimism: weight is lifting, dissolving, shifting, opening up to new considerations

Realization: This is my journey; I am choosing to trust the process.

Catalysts and Impediments:

Potential Pitfalls: yielding to fear, flawed premises, and conditioning (habit patterns of the mind) halts the progress

Catalysts to growth: allowing, disarming, putting down the sword; accepting the (previously) unacceptable, including both self-acceptance and acceptance of the situation

Exercise/Meditation: accepting/disarming: Nothing happened, or did everything happen?

CHAPTER 5

Emerging—Birthing The New

This chapter documents the fifth phase: emergence, bringing forth what is within you, a new way of being and relating to our reality. It involves acknowledging what is here and embracing the present, exactly as it is. With deeper awareness, we can willingly accept the labor pains in this birthing process. With enhanced skills and new insights, we begin breaking ground and laying new tracks into the life we are consciously choosing.

"This is my journey and I am choosing to trust the process."
EXCERPT FROM CASE STUDY

NO MUD, NO LOTUS

Like a gorgeous lotus flower, tender and strong, blossoming up through the mud and gloom, the experience of emergence can only be precisely described in metaphor. It is that uniquely personal. It's as if all the pain that has come before has somehow been perfectly composted to support this bursting forth into new life. The deeper and more painful our suffering and struggle, the more exquisitely we will feel a sense of freedom on the other side of it. We know now from direct experience that we can regard the process of life as a process of giving birth to new dimensions of ourselves, never taking any stage as the final stage, never giving up on life or on ourselves.

What we are bringing forth is simply what was in us all along, deep in our roots, in the form of our human spiritual potential. We had come up against what ancient yogis called the great grinding wheel of life; but rather than being worn down, shredded, and crushed by it, we have held our ground, becoming polished and honed instead. So it's not only about loss, after all. It's about our innate ability to transform difficulty into opportunity for growth, to become strong enough to transcend and include all that has happened in the crucible of our life. It's about the alchemy of converting all this bloody detritus into pure gold, and giving birth to ourselves again and again and again.

> *Deep in their roots*
> *All flowers keep the light.*
> THEODORE ROETHKE

Of the three aspects in the emergence phase, the first involves consciously embracing the present, acknowledging what is still left, still here, and building on those gifts, strengths, and experiences. The second involves managing the labor pains of the birthing process, and this is no easy task. Cycles of relapse into less evolved ways of being, as well as waves of resistance, continue to present themselves. But they are met with ever growing awareness and skill. The third aspect involves actively and diligently manifesting our new way of being until it becomes second nature to us. Here is where we continue to break ground and lay new tracks into the future we are co-creating. This is an important time for courageous action, honest reflection, learning from inevitable setbacks, and receiving the benefits of helping relationships. Realistic expectations and self-compassion are crucial as well. It takes some focus and some hard work to become all that we can be, but ask yourself, what is more important?

"I'm no longer afraid. I know I'm going to be OK somehow.
Things will work out one way or another. I can grow from
this. I can see there is a silver lining to this cloud."
EXCERPT FROM CASE STUDY

EMBRACING THE PRESENT

There's a now famous story about violinist **Itzhak Perlman** that relates to the question of embracing present and doing our best with what is here, even when it is far less than ideal. Perlman was halfway into his solo performance of a major symphonic piece at Lincoln Center when one of his four violin strings suddenly snapped. It was well understood by his audience that to complete a symphonic piece with only three strings would probably not be possible. They fully expected to see him end the performance and slowly exit the stage in his familiar, inimitable manner, on leg braces from childhood polio, ever a model of humility and self-acceptance.

However, he enthralled his audience by doing what was actually considered impossible. Right on the spot, he somehow managed to transpose the entire piece in his head and began playing it masterfully on the only three strings he had. Perlman performed the piece with passion right through to the end and received a standing ovation from his a stunned audience. When asked how he was able to do the inconceivable, his answer was this: "You know, sometimes it is the artist's task to find out how much beautiful music he can still make with what little he has left."

Making something beautiful happen with what little we have left may not be our first instinct in the face of irrevocable loss, but it may be our most evolved instinct. It requires wholeheartedly embracing the present moment—showing up for it, calm and clear, and giving it our best shot with courage, humility, and generosity of spirit, no matter what, regardless of whatever is missing and whatever is still left. This can only happen once we've made real progress in accepting reality as it is, not as we expected it would be. We have all been conditioned to hold certain expectations that will never be met.

Resistance to accepting reality is the glue that keeps suffering in place, arresting our development, and draining our energy. We are prone to having an aversion to what is here and craving what is not here, meanwhile ignoring the opportunity that is actually present, here and now. It is a radical act to give oneself permission to fully appreciate each moment, something to strive for that is both healing and instantly rewarding. Now is the time to discover what is already and always here.

We must be willing to let go of the life we've planned,
so as to have the life that is waiting for us.
JOSEPH CAMPBELL

HERE AND NOW

Consciously choosing where to direct our attention will have a massive impact on how we relate to ourself, others, and to everything that has and will happen in our life. As we have said, it is in exercising our power to choose that we determine who we are. Recognizing this can be enormously encouraging. One very practical and liberating insight of the Buddhist perspective is its teaching on the impermanence of all things, including every thought, emotion, sensation, etc.

It does seem fairly obvious, yet this is something we tend to overlook. Everything that has the nature to arise will also cease. Deepening our understanding and awareness of impermanence and the continual flow of thought leads to greater equanimity by making unhelpful, negative thoughts easier to let go of, harder to take too seriously. This in turn leads to increasing degrees of liberation from emotional suffering.

To experience directly one must be aware of oneself
in the process of repetition, of habits,
of words, of sensations.
That awareness gives you an extraordinary freedom,
so that there can be a renewal,
a constant experiencing, a newness.

JIDDU KRISHNAMURTI

Many shifts in perspective become evident to us during the birthing process of the emergence phase. More and more, our perspective shifts as we realize we haven't lost everything. We still have so much to work with and to be grateful for. We are standing on new ground with less focus on what went wrong and more on how lessons learned from our experience might serve us going forward. We have more confidence that we can and will harvest something of value from this pain and find the thread of gold in it.

Resistant and negative automatic thoughts that may have plagued and blocked us in the past have been replaced by more realistic appraisals of the situation. Now that we've connected with helpful, supportive people along the way, we've learned we can ask for help when we need it. If we have been practicing meditation, we have become increasingly skillful at observing when we are dwelling on the negative and then shifting our focus, directing our attention by choice to what is good in our life and going back to focusing on what works. Breathing deeply, we've become more adept at naturally lowering our anxiety to a healthier level.

As a consequence, we're becoming calmer, more stable, less reactive. This tendency to feel more even-keeled is often interrupted by spontaneous moments of unanticipated joy. Our physical energy improves, and our impulse to make healthy choices is getting stronger, inclining us to get enough exercise and rest and to eat more nutritious foods.

From a behavioral standpoint, our ability to make conscious choices is steadily increasing. As a result, we have better impulse control as our ability to self-regulate keeps improving. Spiritually, we are more and more in the present moment, staying aware and staying awake. We realize that we are not alone and that there is even something mythic about this struggle, this journey we are on.

THE BIRTHING PROCESS, FROM THE INSIDE

If you do not bring forth that which is within you,
that which is within you will destroy you.
If you do bring forth that which is within you,
that which is within you will save you.

JESUS, GOSPEL OF THOMAS

How did this emergence phase unfold with the men and women we've been following? Let's start with what they were saying to themselves as they moved through their turning point. We'll follow with some highlights of their stories:

" . . . I'm listening to my intuition now and trusting it. It's a whole new life, a departure from my prior life in a very significant way. I never would have had the courage to do this. Looking back, I was crippled with fear. I would have talked myself out of my dreams. Now I'm becoming who I am, becoming who I want to be." TED

"It was a revelation to me: You can control this situation from the inside by just not paying attention to people's reaction to you. I don't see it (people staring) anymore. My attitude is wonderful. I know that my purpose in life is to live my life in this disfigured way. To LIVE MY LIFE, to finally get it: to listen to intuitive messages and follow them, to just trust and stop panicking. The universe will provide. Just live it. Drop your worries and surrender. You really have to get on that edge and know you have wings to fly." SARAH

"Meditation changes people. I will never betray myself again. It's been empowering, powerful. I am reclaiming my joy. I can trust my intuition. We're being cared for by the universe. I can trust and surrender to the unknown, to a higher power now. I see things differently now. I am building a new life." JANE

"My crisis has been an amazing catalyst to realizing this whole other dimension. I have directly experienced that there are altered states of consciousness, undeniable to me. There's much more than the physical world. Sometimes in the midst of adversity, things break open, and it allows these things to come forward—an aspect of God? Who knows? It's not definable or defined. People said I was never the same." ANNE

"I simply could no longer stay in the marriage. It was just hanging on to a false myth. I've begun to live from a system of spiritual values. I had to move on. I made yoga, which I love, my life's work. It's a growth process that never stops. I'm able to work through the fears. I've created a new way of living and being. There is freedom from deep within. I have a better connection to people, to life." LISA

"You must live life with courage to be who you are. Honestly, no matter the consequences, people who love you and matter to you will love you no matter what. Those who don't are those you don't need to worry about. You will be the object of criticism and hostility, inevitably. Let it go. It's your only chance." PAUL

"I'm on a spiritual journey. Once you get cancer, you realize that nothing is certain in life. It's not a frightening idea, more of a focusing thought. Things would never have happened in my life without the illness, and they have enriched my life a great deal; it's wonderful in its own way. I'm a better person for it." KIM

"I am still singing in the choir, but I need to be in the chair. Still, it's a good experience. I do what I want to do. I don't know why, but I'm not embarrassed. Something is going on with me. I think I don't care what anyone thinks. I am finding happiness everyday, surprising myself, in a good way." CAROL

"People said I look transfigured. I made a change right there: I moved to life. I had a spiritual healing. I experienced a final self-acceptance. I'm on a path." ALISON

"Something happened that was just a spontaneous moment, an opening to that experience of the unborn, like a lightning bolt of completely radical change, of understanding. And just immediately following that, I felt completely out of the context of ordinary consciousness." JONATHAN

"It all started to come together when I attended to my inner self. There are no coincidences. Be where you are. I came to terms with the loss. I made my peace with it. I can live with it. My goal hasn't changed: I will do my best; just the pathway to getting there is different." FRAN

"I realized my life had been preparing me for this. I have to give back now. My journey has come full cycle. I have a higher level of consciousness. I see how much of my life was lived with the weight of the past and future. I am in the present now. It was a remarkable shift, so freeing." PETER

As soon as you trust yourself,
you will know how to live.

GOETHE

BRINGING FORTH—STORIES OF EMERGENCE

Jane began forging a new life, having left her abusive marriage of 28 years. This meant redefining where she would spend what she still had left. She took courses, volunteered in her community, joined a hiking club, made new friends, and basically reinvented her life. Mike got clean, as he likes to say. He completed his AA program and made a life-changing commitment to bring forth his best vision of himself, to become a role model, leading AA workshops for youth, which he has continued to do to this day. Sarah has built an amazing career, teaching seminars in science of mind, plus designing and co-leading international travel adventures for individuals in wheelchairs. She continues dazzle people with infectious joy and courage wherever she goes.

Daniele became a student activist for several humanitarian causes and still devotes a portion of her time to developing programs for survivors of sexual abuse. She is now in her second year of law school and has become an extraordinary amateur belly dancer as well. Laura has occasional setbacks, cycling with rage and blame, but they are briefer and rarer now. Still motivated and enthusiastic, she continues to progress toward emotional freedom and is greatly relieved to be feeling optimistic again. Ted hired a career coach, completed veterinary school, launched his dream career and has never been happier. It was an adjustment for his family, but they've grown in the process too, which was a good thing for everyone.

Carol's MS has been in remission for several years now, and she is leading a remarkably fulfilling life, taking on new challenges and experiences that she had assumed would be forever beyond her. She now sings regularly with two local choirs. Although she has difficulty standing, they have provided her with a special high stool so she can even perform in concerts at the right height. She participates with huge joy. Kim is in remission as well and still serving as a faculty member at a leading university. She continues to grow personally and professionally and has recently rewritten the nursing school curriculum to include the spiritual needs of cancer patients.

Until we can embrace our lives wholeheartedly,
aware of our limitations and committed to making
the most of our unique circumstances and gifts,
we have not fully accepted ourselves for the people we are
or fully forgiven ourselves for the people we are not.
                              KENT NEWBURN

BRINGING FORTH: THE PROCESS

Giving birth to ourselves is about proceeding with the vision that is within us, even when the territory is unfamiliar, the outcome is uncertain, and the going gets tough. When we think of a chick coming out of its egg, we tend to imagine her all fluffy and perky, which is the exact opposite of how it is in reality. True, the mother usually pecks a few cracks in the shell when she senses it is time, but the heavy work is done by the baby chick, and it's anything but cute.

Trapped, cramped, and gasping for air, the little chick alternates between trying to claw her way out, and collapsing in exhaustion. It takes time. And when she finally makes her way through into the big bright world, she is weary, damp, and naked. Her limp, skinny neck leaning over the broken shell, her head too heavy to lift, tongue hanging out, eyes looking all around, wondering where am I? Labor pains are part of the deal. So if even a chick has to endure some in bringing herself to life, why not we?

You gain strength, experience and confidence
by every experience

where you really stop to look fear in the face.
You must do the thing you cannot do.

ELEANOR ROOSEVELT

VISIONING

Along with the ability to accept and endure some inevitable labor pains, one of the most crucial things to have during the bringing forth phase is a vision of where and how you long to be. **Florence Chadwick** had already distinguished herself by being the first woman to swim across the English Channel. But when she tried to swim to Catalina Island, 15 miles off the coast of California, swimming through icy water, sharks, and dense fog, she gave up only a mile from shore.

Later she said, "I'm not excusing myself, but if I could have seen the land, I might have made it." Two months later, she trained again for the same event, but this time she practiced envisioning the shoreline, just in case a dense fog rolled in, which of course it did. But this time was different. She held an image of land in her mind, which kept her going, straight through the fog, and she persevered till the end. Reaching that shoreline was as much more than a physical accomplishment for Chadwick; it was a spiritual and emotional triumph.

The only thing worse than being blind is having no vision.
Life is either a daring adventure or nothing.
Security is mostly a superstition.
It does not exist in nature.

HELEN KELLER

By the time we make it to the other side, having surpassed our expectations, along with our perceived limitations, we are never the same. We can never be shoehorned into the less evolved person we once were.

No one has said it better than **Eleanor Roosevelt**:

You gain strength, courage, and confidence
by every experience in which you really stop
to look fear in the face.
You are able to say to yourself,
"I have lived through this horror.
I can take the next thing that comes along."
You must do the thing you think you cannot do.

How does it feel, on the inside, to make it to the other side? Paradoxically, we may feel both triumphant and a bit vulnerable the same time. But what is universally experienced is an expanded sense of self, increased confidence and inner strength, deeper connection to others, increased emotional openness and fluidity, and personal authenticity. The key thread running through all of these is crucially significant: greater resilience in the face whatever comes next.

Excerpted directly from case studies during the emergence phase, we can now hear the voice of this resilience in their own words. Here is a **composite** of individuals describing how they have changed and grown in the process:

I'm more able to surrender, to trust the process now,
    to have faith in something, in myself.
I have so little fear now.
I am more able to live in the moment,
    less self-centered, more humble.
I have a heightened sense of connection to all people.
I'm more open to experience.
I have the courage and strength to face whatever I discover.
Only the truth is meaningful.

I don't compare and despair anymore. I'm breaking the chain.
I'm more courageous, more loving, trustworthy,
  more honest with myself and others.
I'm a good friend, a good human being, more sensitive.
I have gratitude. I am more balanced,
and I have more determination.
I've become interested in surrender.
I came to a still point and let it happen.
I'm more connected spiritually. There is no more denial.
My stubbornness was transformed into tenacity.
Fear had kept me back. I had no confidence.
I'm more caring about other people now.
I connect with people more easily. I am more understanding
  with them.
I can listen inside and be guided by intuitive knowing.
You begin to trust your intuition more and more.
You must be willing to listen.
You need willingness to heal, a willingness to let go,
a willingness to examine yourself and your life
and more ability to trust, believe in yourself,
  to trust yourself that you won't lose yourself.
You have more passion for life.
I can honestly step outside myself and
  view the situation with some objectivity.
I can be brutally honest about myself and about everybody
  else.
I see it for what it is, and
I don't make more of it than what it is.
I feel freer and more optimistic.

I'd long been on a spiritual journey but hadn't realized it,
or I had been on it in a way that wasn't productive.
As your life evolves, you need that sense of connectedness,
continuity of life, bring closure to some parts of it, and
really feel them as parts of yourself and build on that.

These statements represent the deepest feelings reported by individuals again and again, echoing the shift in perspective during the process of breaking through and of overcoming.

Self-pity is our worst enemy, and if we yield to it,
we can never do anything wise in this world.
Although the world is full of suffering,
it is full also of the overcoming of it.
HELEN KELLER

MANIFESTATION

This part of emergence involves grounding insights with actions, forging new directions, and laying new tracks into the life that is waiting for us. This is where the proverbial rubber meets the road, because without a plan of action all our good intentions can easily vaporize.

True, sometimes turning points can appear to occur spontaneously, but even then, much has happened beforehand to prepare us for them. Insights, awareness, and continued development of our strengths through self-observation and mindfulness practice will serve to support the process of bringing forth more and more of who we have the potential to be.

OBSTACLES TO EMERGENCE: POTENTIAL PITFALLS

There are multiple potential pitfalls on our way through emergence to the manifestation phase:

- Resistance to letting go of the past minimizes progress.
- Inability to tolerate uncertainty brings us to a halt.
- The momentum of old ways pulls us back.
- Anxiety about not being up to the challenge stunts our growth.
- Fear of failure (or of success) limits our options.
- There is a lack of imagination, a vision, or a dream to energize us.
- Failure to recognize and embrace birthing as creative way to live your life.

As long as we remain aware of these common problems, we can prepare to meet them with skillful anticipation. They may challenge us but they will not derail us. Laying new tracks into the future involves charting new courses of action and ways of being and then repeating those choices until they become new habit patterns, our new default positions. It's about grounding insights into action steps that we can realistically take on a day-to-day basis. This includes working consciously with our old mental programming and replacing negative thoughts with positive statements, like a devoted gardener clearing out weeds. Self-confidence grows each time we risk taking a manageable new step. Positive visualizations enable us to embrace each step in the new direction that we have consciously chosen.

QUESTIONS FOR GROUNDING INSIGHTS INTO ACTIONS

What are three action steps that you can take during the next week to bring forth the best that is within you?

1.＿＿＿＿＿＿＿＿＿＿＿＿＿＿＿＿＿＿＿＿＿＿＿＿＿

2.＿＿＿＿＿＿＿＿＿＿＿＿＿＿＿＿＿＿＿＿＿＿＿＿＿

3.＿＿＿＿＿＿＿＿＿＿＿＿＿＿＿＿＿＿＿＿＿＿＿＿＿

As an irrigator is guiding water to his fields,
as an archer is aiming an arrow,
as a carpenter is carving wood,
the wise are shaping their lives.

BUDDHA

OVERCOMING OBSTACLES

1. Resistance to letting go of the past minimizes progress.

Be not the slave of your own past—
plunge into the sublime seas.
Dive deep and swim far
so you shall come back with self respect,
with new power, with an advanced experience
that shall explain and overlook the old.

RALPH WALDO EMERSON

- Why am I letting the past cheat me out of one more minute of my present and future freedom?
- In theory, can I let it go?
- Could someone else let it go?

2. Inability to tolerate uncertainty brings us to a halt

The psychic task which a person
can and must set for himself
is not to feel secure,
but to tolerate insecurity.

ERICH FROMM

- What emotion am I feeling right now?
- Where in my physical body am I feeling the contraction of fear or heaviness of sorrow?
- Can I try breathing into the area deeply, allowing this tension to be released, restoring my equilibrium?

3. The momentum of old ways of being is pulling us back.

We are always torn between the wish to regress to the womb
and the wish to be fully born.
Every act of birth
requires the courage to let go of something.
ERIC FROMM

- What do I need to transcend now in order to move forward?
- When can I allow this growth to happen?
- Why does it matter?

4. Anxiety about not being up to the challenge stunts growth.

No one can make you feel inferior without your consent.
The future belongs to those who believe in the beauty of their dreams.
You must do the thing you think you cannot do.
ELEANOR ROOSEVELT

- When have I ever felt unequal the task?
- How has that feeling gotten in my way?
- Would I rather continue feeling this way?
  Or would I rather be free?

5. Fear of failure (or of success) limits our options.

Mistakes are the portals of discovery.
JAMES JOYCE

*What lies behind us and before us are small matters
compared to what lies within us.*
RALPH WALDO EMERSON

- What natural strengths and innate capacities have I not been fully using?
- Which personal qualities do I feel most grateful for having?
- Where will I find the courage to proceed?

6. There is a lack of imagination, a vision, or a dream to energize us.

*No pessimist ever discovered the secret of the stars,
or sailed to an uncharted land,
or opened a new doorway for the human spirit.*
HELEN KELLER

- What is my best vision of myself?
- What am I living for?
- And what is keeping me from living wholeheartedly for it?

7. Failure to recognize and embrace birthing as creative way of life

*Only birth can conquer death—
Within the soul, within our lives, there must be—
if we are to experience long survival—*

a continuous "recurrence of birth" to nullify
the unremitting recurrences of death.

JOSEPH CAMPBELL

* What has to die off in order for me to give birth to the next phase of my life?
* If not now, when?
* Again, most importantly, why does it matter?

LIVING SCULPTURE

When the sculptor Michelangelo was asked how he could have possibly carved his masterpiece, the statue of David, out of a rough slab of solid marble, he said he simply carved away everything nonessential to reveal the incredible beauty that was hidden inside all along. This is another apt metaphor for manifesting human potential. Think of your life as a living piece of sculpture that you are constantly shaping and reshaping through your attention and your actions.

We have a sacred opportunity in this very life to bring forth the best vision of ourselves that we can possibly imagine. The first step is to place our primary focus wholeheartedly on what already works in our life. As our positive aspects naturally become strengthened in this, we can more easily transform our negative tendencies, some of which will simply fall away on their own. Carl Jung believed that we have a natural gradient toward wholeness. As many have observed, our future depends on many things, but mostly on us.

In the long run, we shape our lives and we shape ourselves.
The process never ends until we die, and the choices that
we make are ultimately our responsibility.

ELEANOR ROOSEVELT

In the end is it those who have become increasing able tolerate uncertainty and insecurity, particularly in the current absence of old escapes and negative defenses, who will have the wherewithal to proceed. They are the ones who have developed the grit to relinquish control while accepting and enduring the unavoidable labor pains of growth as they forge a new way of being.

They are the ones who have learned how to create a sense of safety from the inside out, trusting the process, walking the walk, day by day and, breath by breath, becoming equal to the task through their own diligent efforts while, at the same time, surrendering to the great mystery in which we are all held.

Everyone suffers, but they are the ones who have suffered in service of growth. They are the ones who actually come to the harvest, more liberated, resilient, wise, and loving than they ever were before. They have not suffered in vain. The insight and wisdom they have acquired can never be taken away. Having experience this, they can never be diminished.

Adversity is the raw material of indestructible happiness.
BUDDHIST TEACHING

Contradictory as this statement may seem, it is so profoundly true. Indeed, it is often through encountering our worst defeats and most formidable obstacles that we come home to ourselves with a level of self-esteem and inner peace that we could not have acquired any other way. It is then that we are ready to bring forth what is in us, the best in us.

There is something waiting inside you,
like an unplayed melody in a flute
RAINER MARIA RILKE

Now is the time to listen deeply for the sound of our own music, our own inner voice, time to combine our capacity for self-reflection with our capacity for action, in accordance with our best vision of ourselves. This is the time for grounding insights into practical steps that carry us forward with steady momentum, through the birthing process. Yes, something in us is dying, but something else is being born, being transformed into something so precious and indestructible that we can only feel mystified and grateful that this is finally, slowly happening.

Emergence is an exercise in inner befriending, in tenacity, self-honoring, and self-loyalty, sometimes against all odds, including our own internal impediments that would otherwise keep us stuck. Sometimes it's an exercise in loving ourselves enough to let go of whatever is toxic for us, be it an attitude, a mind-set, a substance, a relationship, a habit. Can you recognize which patterns having been getting in your way, leading to even subtle forms of self-betrayal? Can you honor yourself enough to practice letting them go?

> *Many people die with their music still in them.*
> *Why?*
> OLIVER WENDELL HOLMES

Freedom from inner obstacles is hard won. It's like hacking through the bushes that separate us from the river of life. We just need to trust the process and stay awake. As Maslow once said, "You will either step forward into growth, or you will step back into safety."

Only we get to choose, again and again and again.

> *The breeze at dawn has secrets to tell you*
> *don't go back to sleep*
> *You must ask for what you really want*
> *don't go back to sleep*

People are going back and forth across the doorsill
where the two worlds touch
The door is round and open
don't go back to sleep

RUMI

EXERCISE: CATALYZING EMERGENCE

Here are some profoundly important questions to **revisit** now, questions to live our life with:

- If you woke up tomorrow magically cured of all your inner obstacles, limitations, and hesitations, free to be all you can be ... how would you know?
- How would you be feeling physically? emotionally? energetically?
- What would you do be doing?
- What actions would you be likely to take?
- What would be different about you?

EXERCISE/MEDITATION: STEPS IN VISUALIZING YOUR BEST SELF

I. Think of a time in your past when you amazed yourself in some very positive way. Maybe you exceeded your own expectations in a challenging situation, or maybe you discovered that you were deeply admired by someone you value, or maybe you just woke up on an ordinary day feeling very happy to be alive, for no particular reason. In any case, you were experiencing yourself with robust sense of joy and self-esteem. Consciously choose to think of this reflection as both your best self and your natural state.

2. Now take a moment to get really comfortable in a quiet, safe space where you won't be disturbed and begin to come home to your body by taking a few deep cleansing inhales and slow, full letting-go exhales. Feel your back relaxing against the back of the chair and then release

the weight of your body into the chair as you begin to let go a little more, allowing your muscles to soften. Savor this moment of effortlessness, just being, just breathing, nothing more. Notice how good this feels as your body relaxes a little more and your mind follows, becoming calmer as you bring your focus to the flow of the breath.

3. Next, invite an image to form of yourself, right here and now, having grown in the process of learning and healing. Imagine yourself facing the biggest challenge that lies ahead for you, one that is most significant and in some way intimidating. See yourself standing on solid ground, feeling calm and relaxed, safe and strong, with a sense of patient anticipation.

4. Now invite the energy of your best self, as you remembered it in Step 1, and visualize that positive energy filling your entire being, mind, body and spirit. See yourself in your natural state, infused with a sense of optimism and unwavering confidence. Welcome whatever positive images come to mind, including any metaphors that may occur to you, images that represent to you a sense of endurance, forging through the forest, hacking away at the obstacles that separate you from the river of life, the hero's journey. See yourself meeting the challenge at hand with your best self, triumphant. You, the hero of your own story.

And I have the firm belief in this now,
not only in terms of my own experience,
but in knowing about the experience of others,
that when you follow your bliss, doors will open where
you would not have thought there were going to be doors,
and where there wouldn't be a door for anybody else.
JOSEPH CAMPBELL

SUMMARY POINTS: CHAPTER 5:
EMERGING—BIRTHING THE NEW

Cognition: I haven't lost everything. I still have _____.

Premise: I can harvest something valuable from this pain; I can find the thread of gold in this.

NAT → RRR: I can awaken into the present moment at any time; I can ask for help when I need it (the conscious RRRs balance the NATs).

Emotions: calmer, more stable; more time in neutral, with spontaneous moments of unanticipated joy

Physical: energy improves; new impulses to maintain optimum wellness: nutrition, exercise, rest

Behavioral: increasing ability to make conscious choices; resistance decreases, greater impulse control, greater ability to self-regulate

Spiritual: staying aware, staying awake, more time in the present moment

Realization: This is my journey; I am choosing to trust the process.

Realization: I am not alone; there is even something mythic in this struggle.

Catalysts and Impediments:

Potential Pitfalls: inability to tolerate uncertainty, resistance to letting go of past; pain in the absence of old comfort; fear of not being up to the challenge

Catalysts to growth: increased ability to endure labor pains; growing of new way of being; developing new external and internal sources of safety

Exercise/Meditation: visualizing self as enduring, forging through the forest, for example, making headway toward the river of life, coming home to oneself

Adversity is the raw material
of indestructible happiness
Buddhist teaching

CHAPTER 6

Integrating—Permanent Traits

This chapter elucidates the sixth phase, integration. It is a time of empowered action and assimilation of new levels of conscious awareness. Our raw experience has been distilled into a quality of wisdom, understanding, and optimism that previously eluded us. Our inner strength is deepened, our perspective broadened.

We can observe in ourselves greater resilience and emotional freedom, increasing autonomy, and wholeness. We have moments of feeling gratefully immersed in our new way of being. Skills enhanced during earlier phases continue to serve us in self-motivating ways. More and more, we see evidence that we are becoming who we were meant to be.

"Now I am uniquely equipped to handle whatever lies ahead. My life can have new meaning, not just in spite of what happened but ironically, because of how I have handled what happened"

EXCERPT FROM CASE STUDY

This is a time of action, taking very deliberate new steps and diligently practicing specific ways of being, based on our newly acquired insights. Three areas of focus during the integration phase are immersion, motivation, and self-observation. It's about composting all the negativity of the past—defeat, adversity, loss, sorrow, etc.—and transforming it into the fuel that carries us forward.

This is, at its essence, the ultimate creative act of our precious human life. It enables us to transcend the past while day by day bringing us into alignment with our true purpose. To say it is of supreme importance is an understatement. Some say it is what we came here to do. Ultimately, it's about actualizing our potential and fulfilling our destiny.

Our duty as people is to proceed as if
limits to our ability did not exist.
We are collaborators in creation.
PIERRE THEILLARD DE CHARDIN

IMMERSION

During the immersion phase, we actually do consistently become what we practice being. By taking deliberate new steps into unfamiliar directions, we are establishing a future way of being based on conscious choice. It is exciting one minute, terrifying the next, and requires loyalty to our best vision, a practical strategy for progressing, and enough skill in stress-reduction tools to help stay the course. Again, cultivating mindfulness as we go provides ever-increasing resilience in the face of uncertainty. This is how it was experienced by some of the individuals we've been tracking in earlier chapters. Their comments read like a practical blueprint, once again mapping out the territory of emergence in the transformative experience.

Live by longing, and endure:
summon a vision and declare it pure.
THEODORE ROETHKE

"My biggest lesson? You have to be more awake for these transforming moments, not just the great big earth-shaking ones. I can now see smaller ones that present themselves as opportunities in everyday life that I would never have noticed before. Nothing is permanent. Life takes on a different dimension, and instead of this having a frightening quality, it takes on an amazing array of opportunities. I'm operating on a different level of conscious awareness." KIM

"I've just got to go out there every day and live this truth, this authentic self, this universal truth, and just blow people away by just doing that, by actually living it. My disability is not in the way anymore. I can go wherever I want. Who cares how this looks to anybody? Their opinion is not my business. It is so freeing. I have never been happier. My heart opened up. There are only two emotions: love and fear. Love flows, fear blocks." SARAH

"I've been so blessed, it's time to give back. We have to carry each other for a long, long time. If they hadn't carried me, I'd be dead. I have really been to hell and back suffering with this addiction. I've been to the extreme bottom. I met the crossroad and made the right decision. We do have the ability to think and choose." MIKE

"It's given me an incredible amount of compassion for people striving for their victory. It is a quest of facing myself more and more honestly, and there are many more layers below the onion skin. I don't feel afraid of things falling apart. In meditation, my faith that I'm okay is confirmed. It takes time, but it's all worth it." JANE

"I had really believed that I was a pretty useless human being, devoid of talent, unable to accomplish anything. I had such low self-esteem. I was unlovable really. It's been a major transformation. I am more confident every day. I am thriving in my new life, living life differently, happy to be alive." LISA

"The spiritual awakening that's happening in individuals is just a reflection of what is happening on a global level. The earth itself is a spiritual being undergoing a transformation itself, and we are all just points of consciousness within that spiritual being. We are all, more or less, part of this human evolution." PETER

"It hasn't been one dimensional; it's multifaceted. It's caused a lot of change in me in many different areas. I had neglected my spiritual side. Being able to really empathize with people matters. I've been opened up in ways that I wouldn't have allowed myself to be before. I've cranked myself wide open, expanded myself, loosened the grip on my need to be in control. I've lightened up! I always thought, later. Later is now!" FRAN

"You have to be able to give yourself up to it in order to have it. You can go over the cliff in that boat, but you're going to be all right. There is self-acceptance. I am on a spiritual path. I practice meditation every day. I am different now, very peaceful, sometimes blissful. I'd never really surrendered before. Now letting go is a way of life." ALISON

"Trusting is key, really feeling that there is a path, and in order to honor it you have to trust your intuition. I'm okay now with the unexpected twists and turns. I even seek them out. Sometimes they seem completely out of character to me, but I honor them now and trust that they will lead me to where I should go. They have!" DANIELE

IMMERSION AND SELF-SOOTHING: STAYING ON TRACK

Mindfulness enhances the chances of staying on course for many reasons. For starters, it expands our awareness and opens our inner space for the possibility of practicing certain spiritual strengths and stress management skills when we most need them. Skill at self-soothing, e.g., is regarded as an important indicator of an individual's overall mental well-being, as well as one's ability to manage stressful situations without coming un-glued and derailed. It is a key component of resilience and a crucial factor in the trajectory of our own emergence.

The farther along we proceed on the journey, the more adept we need to become at what psychologists call self-soothing. It begins with mindful awareness and breathing. This, in turn, leads to higher levels of both emotional intelligence and physical well-being, as we discussed in Chapter 1 on the Mind-Body Matrix.

It is enormously helpful to increase skillfulness in this area. Our ability to maintain equanimity can be steadily enhanced during the process of emergence and maintained throughout our entire life. There is no end to our growth in this strength. Through mindfulness of our physical state, we can observe levels of agitation and anxiety early in the game, before they get hold of us.

Through deep breathing, we can observe and then shift, in three to five slow deep breaths, as our body begins to release tension, feeling more grounded and at ease. As we calm our body, we calm our mind. Like clear water flowing down a mountain creek once branches are removed, calming energy flows freely and easily in our body, all on its own, once excess tensions have been released.

The space created in that moment is potentially transformational because it gives us the distance we need to liberate ourselves from reactive thinking and behavior, the nemesis of growth. It's simply a matter of practice. If we have the intention and are willing to practice, we can become more and more adept at this. As we have discussed, when our mind and body are calmer, we have fullest access to both our emotional intelligence, our most rational thinking and our intuitive wisdom. Every time we practice a new, more conscious way of being, we are grooving new neural pathways that support our becoming who we choose to be. We are changing and growing purposefully, in response to intention and repetition.

I wake from sleep, and take my waking slow.
I learn by going where I need to go.
THEODORE ROETHKE

Practicing mindfulness and developing equanimity also lead us to feel happier and more comfortable in the present while allowing us to move forward into our future, the one we have imagined for ourselves. Mindfulness enhances emotional intelligence, enabling us to be more responsive and aware in general, more able to set healthy boundaries, to be self-protective when necessary, to be selective in our choices, etc. Mindfulness is a win, win, win, win, win.

We are shaped and fashioned by what we love
GOETHE

What do you truly love? Where and how do you long to be in this world, despite everything that has happened and has failed to happen? In one of her most tender and poignant poems *Wild Geese*, **Mary Oliver** reaches out to us:

Whoever you are, no matter how lonely,
the world offers itself to your imagination,
calls to you like the wild geese, harsh and exciting—
over and over announcing your place
in the family of things.

In her most compelling poem, *A Summer Day*, Oliver reminds us of "one wild and precious life":

Tell me, what else should I have done?
Doesn't everything die at last, and too soon?
Tell me, what is it you plan to do
with your one wild and precious life?

MOTIVATION DURING THE INTEGRATION PHASE

As many experts have observed, action often **precedes** motivation. It's not the other way around. Progress itself fuels motivation, and steady progress soon becomes self-sustaining. Thanks to our brain's neuroplastic ability to naturally morph in response to repeated behaviors, positive actions become more ingrained. Meanwhile, negative habit patterns and impulses that once ruled over us are becoming weaker and weaker in the process and gradually fading away.

Through increased awareness and repetition, new chosen ways of being eventually become permanent traits. In the process of learning, change and growth, whether we are learning a new skill or a new way of being in the world, we move through four distinct phases on our way to self-mastery:

1. unconscious incompetence
2. conscious incompetence
3. conscious competence
4. unconscious competence   [mastery]

We are rewarded as we go, with glimpses of our undiscovered self that will delight and amaze us, giving us enough courage and optimism to endure. Our strength grows with each conscious choice and deliberate action that represents growth. The bigger the obstacle, the more glorious the experience of triumphing over it. Practice being what you want to be, here and now. Your job here is not to critique your rate of progress but to last in it, to not get discouraged.

Even if our efforts of attention seem for
years to be producing no result,
one day a light that is in exact proportion
to them will flood the soul.

SIMONE WEIL

Despite whatever setbacks occur, never turn your back on yourself. Just trust the process and hold on to your best vision of how you can be. Mindfulness enhances the chances of staying on course as we practice continuously letting go of negativity (fear, resentment, rigidity, inertia) and bringing ourselves back into the present moment where our opportunity for growth lies waiting.

Heaven and hell are not places one goes after death,
but in the here and now!
The gates of heaven and hell will open to you at any time.

HAKUIN

Let's take a quick look at what factors would constitute the gates of hell, all of which represent the now familiar barriers to development. Then we'll look at the exciting part: the gates to heaven. There's nothing better for recharging our motivation and informing our sense of direction than to take a closer look at these lists of personal qualities with an eye toward where we see ourselves in them. In order to bring forth our best going forward, what do we need more of? What do we need less of? Catalysts and impediments to transformation, as observed by psychologists and psychiatrists interviewed in my research, shed further light on the process of transformation.

PROFESSIONAL OBSERVATIONS ON TRANSFORMATIVE GROWTH

At this point, I'd like to summarize the conclusions drawn by the professionals as they are the voice of direct experience over many years. Their voices are most encouraging and informative as they lay out both the obstacles and the catalysts to transformation for us here. May their words of wisdom and insight galvanize your motivation to proceed with courageous energy.

IMPEDIMENTS: FEAR, AVOIDANCE, RIGIDITY

According to the professionals I interviewed regarding this critical stage in the process, the following traits were named as the most common forms of *resistance to growth*:

1. Inability to assume responsibility for the self, while projecting blame onto others
2. Holding on to old patterns of response or outmoded ways of looking at the world
3. Unwillingness to risk trying something different
4. Excessive need for safety
5. Intolerance for uncertainty
6. Susceptibility to others' disapproval
7. Obsessive stance, rigidity
8. Holding on to anger
9. Inability to relinquish control
10. Close-mindedness
11. Unresolved past issues
12. Self-worth issues

Underlying all of these obstacles to change is the presence of a pervasive sense of fear, which is often unacknowledged or unconscious. Bringing disowned fears to consciousness is a prerequisite for working through them. The problem is that we are often so embedded in our illusions that we are unable to discern their presence. Meanwhile, these illusions, filters, amplifications, and unconscious biases are shaping and limiting our perception of our options and ourselves in insidious ways.

As a consequence, there is an ongoing need for self-investigation, self-confrontation, and courageous, compassionate support, especially when it feels like one part of us would rather stay trapped in a cocoon while another part of us is longing to spread its wings. We feel the opposing instincts of life and death in conflict within us.

This is the ego-cide concept discussed earlier, where an aspect of the individual needs to die off in order for the next level of individuation in a higher level of consciousness to emerge. This has also been described in the shamanic tradition as the initiation born out of the depths of your symbolic death. The ego-cide concept is echoed in the testimonies of the transformed individuals interviewed in this research. The dynamic of crisis and emergence involves a period of decline and of falling apart as a prelude to rebirth in a higher consciousness.

By daily dying, I have come to be.
THEODORE ROETHKE

From the professional's viewpoint, the turning point is actually the point of breaking open, where the defenses that have held change at bay for so long, have now begun to crumble. The individual has an awareness of being in the most extreme difficulty, and often there is an experience of actually being shocked out of old patterns, forced by circumstances out of them. The critical mass notion is operating here. It is often acknowledged that earlier warning signals that change was necessary had been disregarded or missed altogether, sometimes for years on end.

Resistance to change and fear of the unknown work against us at this point. Few of us are really prepared to listen to and act on the first intuitive messages of this kind. This "unconsciousness" may be attributable to the habit patterns of the mind that interfere with our seeing reality as it is. This includes the deeply ingrained outmoded attitudes and limiting beliefs that have been tenaciously getting in the way all along. In any case, the next critical component in the process of transformation is a certain willingness to take the impulse seriously, a readiness to take the leap of faith. Joseph Campbell has a word for it: "Jump!" And now, the good news.

CATALYSTS: RESILIENCE, FLEXIBILITY, AUTONOMY

On the flip side, the professionals listed the most frequently observed attributes seen as *key factors* in the *process of profound change*. According to the experts I interviewed, whenever these qualities were present in individuals, they were bound to amaze themselves as their stories unfolded in remarkably life-affirming ways. These are the very qualities that make turning points both possible and probable on the journey toward a more highly evolved way of being.

EXERCISE: FOCUSING ON QUALITIES FOR MEANINGFUL CHANGE

1. Willingness to examine oneself
2. Readiness to let in advice and new information
3. Perseverance, self-determination, optimism
4. Past experience in meeting challenges effectively
5. Readiness to being different from how one has always been
6. Willingness to change
7. Opening to a higher consciousness
8. Sense of hopefulness
9. Increased self-awareness
10. Ability to trust intuitive insight
11. Sufficient sense of security
12. Ability to tolerate self-confrontation
13. Ability to risk being true to oneself

The last two were seen as absolutely crucial to enabling individuals to get past the hurdles and evolve into becoming more of who they really are in their full authenticity. An underlying theme common to each of these strengths is essentially the quality of relative fearlessness. What's critical here is not the absence of fear but the ability to manage fear effectively enough to get past it and really grow, which is what transformation evidently hinges on.

Many of these qualities point to having the strength to shake off the ego-alien parts of the self and assume greater authenticity. According to the professionals I interviewed, the ability to transform seems to center on honest and courageous confrontation, flexibility and openness to change, openness to the creative/spiritual impulse, and an ability to let go of limiting beliefs. The developmental process often involves the ability to mourn a loss (of a hope or a dream, as well as a more tangible loss) and complete the grieving process before one can proceed to the next level. It demands a willingness to surrender—a readiness to break down and break apart in order to move into an expanded level of conscious awareness.

SELF-OBSERVATION DURING THE INTEGRATION OF INNER CHANGE

Surely the one thing which can bring about
a fundamental change,
a creative, psychological release,
is everyday watchfulness,
being aware from moment to moment of our motives,
the conscious as well as the unconscious.
JIDDU KRISHNAMURTI

How does it feel when we've made it through to the integration phase? Edifying and gratifying, among other things. One of the many rewards of the journey thus far is that most of us have become increasingly self-observant and self-aware in the process of working mindfully through the previous stages.

There is the realization that we are uniquely equipped to handle what comes next in a more conscious and skillful manner. A frequently expressed sentiment is that "my life can have new meaning, not just in spite of what happened but, ironically, because of how I have been able to deal with what happened."

COGNITIVELY There is the recognition that this new reality is workable, along with a certain confidence in facing what's ahead. Having survived the wild emotional storms of the earlier phases, we now know from experience that our ship is seaworthy and that, clearly, we are evolving. In contrast to earlier, limited and negative assumptions that kept us in patterns of avoidance and stagnation, our new premise is exhilarating and forward-moving: "This challenge can serve me."

Instead of backing away from change, we observe ourselves embracing the unknown with the understanding that we can continue to become stronger, wiser, and more alive. No longer viewing uncertainty with fear, we can now regard it as our *growing edge*, our next developmental task to be met and mastered, trusting that we can continue to elevate our life though conscious, deliberate, meaningful endeavors.

We've become more adept at replacing NATs (negative automatic thoughts) with RRRs (rational realistic responses). We see that we are much more than our past suffering and our old limiting perspectives. On good days, which come more and more often, we know that we are pure potentiality, in the process of healing, learning, and growth—in the process of transforming, of becoming more realistic and more conscious.

More and more, this clarity of thinking prevails. Negative thought patterns gradually weaken and fade. Our brain is continually reshaping itself in response to each repetition of every beneficial action, emotion, and thought, making it increasingly easy to stay on track.

EMOTIONALLY AND PHYSICALLY From an emotional standpoint, we are in a very good place. Old constricted feelings of helplessness, sadness, and dread have been replaced with a new sense of gratitude and expansiveness. We are experiencing new levels of inner peace and joy, as well as heightened awareness. Feelings of compassion and loving kindness toward ourselves and others have become a common occurrence. Physically, our energy has improved, and our tendency to maintain optimum wellness is getting easier and easier. We're sleeping better and finding it easier to follow through on getting sufficient exercise and nutrition.

BEHAVIORALLY AND SPIRITUALLY From a behavioral standpoint, we notice an increasing ability to make conscious choices in service of growth. Socially, we are becoming more connected to ourselves and others, more cooperative, and more collaborative. We are becoming a spiritual warrior, capable of staying aware and awake in the present moment.

We are increasingly mindful, balanced, flexible, discerning, compassionate, confident, tender-hearted, resilient, and brave. Our most important and sustaining realization is, "I have surpassed my own expectations of myself; I am uniquely equipped to meet new challenges and serve others."

SKILLFULNESS BECOMES INTEGRATED We've become increasingly skillful at identifying and handling potential pitfalls. We understand that we all have occasional regressive tendencies that inevitably cause setbacks. With awareness and mindfulness, we recognize and release fear early in the game, while it is more manageable.

We renew our determination not to yield to the pull of old habit patterns, and we remain committed to exercising discipline in resisting these regressive tendencies. We maintain self-command, from moment to moment, day by day, catalyzing our forward momentum. We keep laying down new tracks, new neural pathways through diligent effort, focused attention, and sheer tenacity.

Transformation is both ordinary and extraordinary. We have had a powerful learning experience on which to build, a touchstone that is our own. Now it's about trusting ourselves, trusting what we've witnessed firsthand. Sometimes it's about having the skills simply to tolerate feeling empty, lost, and alone. Sometimes it's about the reclaiming of formerly denied aspects of the self.

We have an increased ability to be autonomous as we continue to uncover and become more and more of who we really are. It's about becoming more fully alive. It's not just the quality of our life that hinges on this, but the very essence of our life going forward.

JOURNALING EXERCISE: THOUGHTS TO PONDER AND INCUBATE

Take a break for a moment and savor some deep cleansing inhales and slow full exhales. Then read each of the following quotes, noticing how they make you feel. Then ask yourself this question, and write your responses in a journal.

How does each of these three statements relate specifically in my life?

I

*People seldom see
the halting and painful steps by which
even the most insignificant success is achieved.*

ANNE SULLIVAN

2

*The important thing is this:
to be able at any moment
to sacrifice what you are
for what you could become.*

CHARLES DU BOIS

3
If we all did what we are capable of doing,
we would truly astound ourselves.
THOMAS EDISON

SUMMARY POINTS: CHAPTER 6:
INTEGRATING—PERMANENT TRAITS

"Now I am uniquely equipped to handle whatever lies ahead;
my life can have new meaning –not just in spite of what hap-
pened but because of how I have handled what happened"
EXCERPT FROM CASE STUDY

Cognition: I can work with this reality; my ship is seaworthy, I am evolving.

Premise: This challenge can serve me: I can become stronger, wiser, more alive with this. I can elevate my life through conscious endeavor.

NAT → RRR: I am not my past suffering, my old limiting perspective; I am in the process of transforming, becoming conscious, increasingly realistic. (NB: RRRs dominate thinking as NATs weaken and fade.)

Emotions: sense of inner peace and joy, new gratitude, awareness, loving kindness, compassion, expansiveness

Physical: energy improves; heightened tendency to maintain wellness: nutrition, exercise, rest

Behavioral: increasing ability to make conscious choices; becoming more connected, cooperative, collaborative

Spiritual: spiritual warrior: staying aware, awake, more in the present moment

Realization: I have surpassed my own expectations of myself; I am uniquely equipped to meet new challenges and serve others.

Catalysts and Impediments:

Potential Pitfalls: yielding to fear and the momentum of old ways, regressive tendencies cause inevitable backslides; spiral dynamic

Catalysts to growth: laying down new tracks through diligent effort, tenacity, focus, joyful exertion, discipline in resisting regressive tendencies

EXERCISE/MEDITATION:

If we all did what we are capable of doing
we would truly astound ourselves.

THOMAS EDISON

CHAPTER 7

Evolving—Flourishing

WHOLENESS: AT A HIGHER LEVEL OF CONSCIOUSNESS

This chapter celebrates the seventh phase, flourishing, where we experience ourselves as truly thriving, even in the face of adversity, which, of course, life continues to present in one form or another. We are increasingly in the flow of life, focusing on what has meaning for us as individuals, connecting with friends and loved ones with presence, and sharing our commitment to a higher purpose. We continue to learn and grow, with more resilience, gratitude, and loving kindness, savoring of life's blessings in ways we could not have imagined.

The gift that keeps on giving? It's what we became in the process of transformation that serves us, and everyone we touch, in the end.

"I wish no one had to suffer, but in my case
it was an important catalyst to my growth;
I am more grateful, humble, connected, loving, and
really fearless, etc. than I ever thought possible."
EXCERPT FROM CASE STUDY

We started this book with the heroic story of the botanical artist named **Margot**, whose ultimate response to devastating tragedy was reflected in her further artistic development and personal evolution. She didn't wither or shut down, diminished by loss; she came to life whole-heartedly, passionately. In moving through the phases of transformative growth, her work and her life demonstrated what it's like to transcend and include your history. She was able to compost her loss and broken-ness, embrace unstoppable change, view her crisis as opportunity, and harvest a gift of profound value, enabling her to bring forth a whole new and more evolved way of experiencing life. No doubt, she initially suf-fered painfully and was temporarily immobilized by grief. But in the end, Margot responded to adversity by becoming catalyzed and even galva-nized by it. She is still giving birth to herself in ever new ways, still open-ing to life, truly flourishing. She has now surpassed her previous levels of artistic expression to create a brilliant body of work that might not have existed otherwise. And the world would not have had it.

TRIUMPHANT SPIRIT

We'll end with a very public figure whose life story is compelling in quite a different way: **Olga Bloom**, founder of BargeMusic, a uniquely romantic venue for classical music, moored right below the Brooklyn Bridge. Olga was a young musician performing in New York City when she met a fel-low violinist, Tobias Bloom, with whom she fell madly in love. They mar-ried one week later and spent the next 25 years living happily ever after.

Gathering with friends on the weekends to play chamber music in the intimacy of their beach home, the Blooms lived simply and passionately. They never had children. When Tobias died in 1975, Olga was all alone and absolutely devastated. Their marriage and the passion they shared for music had been her whole life.

She might have given up, allowed her life to narrow down. She could have spent the rest of her years looking through the rearview mirror of her life, stuck in grief for all the irretrievable good times that were over. She could have succumbed to despair for many reasons, as so many people do.

But Olga Bloom did just the opposite. Like Margot and like the many unsung heroes in this book, she moved through the phases of transformation, from grieving to emerging, from breaking down to breaking through. She went on to live an amazing life of unanticipated chapters that both included and transcended her history.

Longing to bring forth in a new form the essence of what she loved most, Bloom decided to create a performance space for classical music that was enchanting and intimate, a place where musicians could develop their artistry and where audiences could fall in love with the experience of being there. She started by mortgaging her house and buying a retired coffee barge for $10,000. From a scrap yard on Staten Island, she retrieved mahogany paneling that had been stripped from junked ferries.

She then applied her knowledge of the acoustical components inside a violin to create fabulous acoustics for the space inside the old barge. Against all odds. But would she ever be taken seriously? Would her dream of a floating concert hall prove feasible, or was it destined to be remembered as a preposterous folly?

She invited young student musicians to begin rehearsing there. They came in droves. When she needed help hooking up to water and electric power, the city of New York and utility companies were so enthralled with this determined little woman and her wild courage that they opened doors for her that would have otherwise remained shut.

Brass sconces installed, Steinway delivered, seating arranged, cookies baked, the word went out, and finally the chamber orchestra was ready to perform. At Bloom's first concert, floating there in the East River in the shade of the Brooklyn Bridge, overlooking the Manhattan skyline, the barge was filled to capacity.

That was 1977. BargeMusic is still going strong, a unique cultural treasure, performing 220 chamber music concerts annually in what has been described as a startlingly beautiful and magical space. A passionate and loyal audience has been flocking to its mooring all these years.

When I first met her after a concert, Olga was in her 80s, surrounded by friends and strangers. Lavished with admiration and affection, roses, and bravas for creating this extraordinary gift to the world, she simply said in response, *"It's been my handrail to sanity."* She was tiny, she was old, but she had a radiance that could light up a room.

Although the others in this book have stories that are less publicly dramatic, they are every bit as transformational in their own way because each of the individuals had hit the proverbial wall or bottom or both. Their lives were at a standstill where the risk of spiraling downward was highly likely, simply the path of least resistance. But each of them woke up in time and fought the good fight.

They gave birth to new and better dimensions of themselves that had not previously existed. They experienced firsthand what it is like to be fired in the alchemist's crucible and to come out golden on the other side. They recreated themselves from the inside out. They experienced what it is like to be fully alive, engaged in the art of living and transforming. We are hard-wired for it.

When the artist is alive in any person,
whatever his kind of work may be,
he becomes an inventive, searching, daring, self-expressive creature.
He becomes interesting to other people.
He disturbs, upsets, enlightens,
and opens ways for better understanding.
Where those who are not artists are trying to close the book,
he opens it and shows there are still more pages possible

ROBERT HENRI

Flourishing is both the endpoint for this model of transformative growth and the starting point for actually living it, sustaining it, after all is said and done. It certainly lacks the drama of the earlier stages, and that's a good thing. At my college graduation, the baccalaureate speaker made the comment that if you think that today marks the end of your education, we have failed you as an institution. He emphasized that the whole purpose was to instill a love of learning and self-education that would continue throughout our entire life. It is my deepest hope that reading this book will contribute in some way to your natural impulse to learn and heal and grow and that you will meet the inevitable crises ahead with enough awareness, courage, and skill to transform them into your next leap forward in your personal evolution.

> *The greatest problems in life can never be solved;*
> *they can only be outgrown.*
> CARL G. JUNG

FLOURISHING AS A WAY OF LIFE

We've been tracking the process of transformation, phase by phase, in individuals' lives. Let's conclude by taking a look at how profoundly they changed by the time they came full cycle to the flourishing phase. How were they different? Were there any commonalities shared by all as they went forward in their respective directions? The answer is yes, with few exceptions. Were they battle weary? Not really.

Across the board, they reported feeling energized and far more confident in themselves than they ever had been before. They tended to feel more grounded and balanced, as if they had been put to the test, a horrifically rough one, and had won the gold medal. They were more self-aware, more mindful of themselves and others, and more deeply grateful.

In the depth of winter, I finally learned that within me
there lay an invincible summer.

ALBERT CAMUS

From a cognitive standpoint, they tended to be fairly philosophical in retrospect about what they had been through. They were able to appreciate how much they had learned about themselves and about life, and most could readily see the positive aspects of their ordeal. They all saw themselves as wiser, and most were more optimistic. Many of them used words like thriving and flourishing to describe their present state.

Some felt that they were in the flow of life for the first time in years or, in some cases, ever. Many were finally experiencing a sense of equanimity, having witnessed the way their intensely negative emotional states had come and gone. In a sense, they truly embodied the Buddhist teaching that no feeling is final. As a result of what they had experienced, most reported that they we were less prone to despair and more inclined to trust life in general.

EMBRACING THE INEVITABLE: ACCEPTANCE AND RESPONSIBILITY

In terms of basic assumptions, a larger perspective and a new premise had gradually replaced their previously limited view. They intimately understood that, while some suffering is unavoidable, it can and does provide motivation for transforming one's life and increasing conscious awareness. Emotional pain can be composted to support and nourish our growth. One of the key markers of emotional maturity is the ability to deal constructively with reality. This involves assuming full responsibility for everything within our power to change, while cultivating full acceptance of all that is truly beyond our control. Denial only delays the inevitable. The goal is to face everything and avoid nothing. This is what it means to be a spiritual warrior.

To be a warrior is not a simple matter of wishing to be one.
It is rather an endless struggle that will go on
to the very last moment of our lives.
Nobody is born a warrior, in exactly the same way
that nobody is born an average man.
We make ourselves into one or the other.

CARLOS CASTANEDA

MEANING AND PURPOSE: FACING THE FUTURE

Another dramatic difference reported by individuals in this study was their change in attitude regarding future challenges. Even among those who were most immobilized by fear in the earlier phases, most of them had replaced their old negative and fearful ways of reacting to crisis with a very different response. They had come feel that, come what may, they had confidence in their ability to handle whatever happens. Having used their personal crisis as a springboard to living more consciously and expansively, they were clearly more optimistic about facing whatever challenges lie ahead.

GIVING BACK

They recognized that they were uniquely qualified to help those facing similar problems, and some made the commitment to use their transformative experience to help others who were oppressed. This was enormously empowering for them. They felt more capable of doing great things and were less inhibited about putting themselves out there. Somewhere in every heart and soul, there is a holy curiosity about what could be. These people were now more in touch with the mystery of their own life.

As a whole, they were kinder, happier, more empathetic, and more loving toward themselves and others. They were grateful for having grown personally. Many reconnected to life's simple pleasures with a new level of involvement and appreciation for friends and family, for music, for nature, etc. Some were actively practicing various forms of healing arts or spiritual practice, such as yoga, meditation, tai chi, drumming, dance, etc. Several reported a new sense of fulfillment through forms of creative expression like writing and visual arts.

> *Creativity is a central source of meaning in our lives ....*
> *and when we are involved in it, we feel that we are living*
> *more fully than during the rest of life.*
>
> MIHALY CSIKSZENTMIHALYI

SELF-TRANSCENDENCE

The happiest and most fulfilled individuals, by their own testimony, experienced a level of self-transcendence that led them to reach out beyond themselves to contribute to a greater cause. Some emphasized that they received more than they gave, noting that the experience of this helping connection deepened the healing process for them while giving their life purpose and meaning. Their efforts now were more for the sake of the whole, and while this helped the world, it completed something within them at the same time.

> *The dedicated life is the life worth living.*
> *You must give with your whole heart.*
>
> ANNE DILLARD

LASTING CHANGES: PERMANENT TRAITS

From a purely physical standpoint, many of the people featured in this book found it easier to remain committed to a healthy lifestyle geared toward optimum wellness and were less prone to succumbing to old negative habits and tendencies. This was very liberating for many. Most found their healthier lifestyle self-motivating. Emotionally, they had become more resilient and stress-hardy across the board, as predicted. Most described their lives as having more balance. From a behavioral standpoint, many believed that they indeed were more constructive, more cooperative and collaborative, and more inclined to see themselves in a larger context.

They had become more humble, less judgmental, more connected, and more compassionate toward others. They had a greater sense of responsibility toward themselves and this gift of life, along with the impulse to honor their unique gifts.

Self-loyalty and autonomy were the threads running though their commitment toward opening to life and bringing forth what had previously remained within them. They were enthused about continuing on the journey of self-discovery, the path of awareness, and the joy of self-expression. They had more positive anticipation and curiosity regarding the future. They were living examples of how the ancient myth of Procrustes can play out in one's life.

RECLAIMING DENIED PARTS OF OURSELVES

In Greek mythology, **Procrustes** was a famous innkeeper on the road to Athens who controlled the gates to the city. Because ancient Athens was a vibrant center of culture, knowledge, commerce, and sophistication, people from the countryside flocked there in hopes of experiencing all it had to offer. However, in order to gain access to the city, each villager had to spend one night at this inn, sleeping on a very specific bed. The Procrustean bed was designed to force conformity to an arbitrary standard established by Procrustes.

If you were too small for the bed frame, your body was torturously stretched on this medieval wooden rack until it fit the standard. If you were too big for the bed, your extremities were hacked off. Equally torturous. Yet the desire to enter into the society of Athens, to fit in and be accepted, was so strong that people tolerated this cruel practice. In the course of growing up, particularly during adolescence and young adulthood, we all spend some time on the Procrustean bed in order to conform to whatever cultural standards and norms we specifically value.

In that process, we acquire certain arbitrary traits that allow us fit in but are not natural to us, nor do they serve us in the end. They get in the way of our living with full autonomy and authenticity. Once we become aware of having some culturally induced traits that were not our natural state to begin with, we can give ourselves permission to let them go. We don't need to remain artificially stretched into areas that lack meaning for us. On the flip side, what about the perfectly natural parts of ourselves that were lobbed off or went underground in the process of fitting in to our particular culture?

Now is the time to remember and reclaim denied parts of ourselves that never quite fit the mold. For that very reason, they may be an untapped source of wholeness for us. Maybe we always longed to play the tuba, even badly. Who knows how much joy, fulfillment, and self-acceptance that could bring to us and to our listeners, who may, thanks to us, feel inspired to be more playful and pursue an avocation despite being a total novice? Maybe we want to make very unusual pottery, in the style of Wabi-Sabi, the celebration of beauty in imperfection. Very juicy. Or we might want to write a poem or sing a song or embrace a worthy cause and bring our uninhibited best to it. There are a thousand ways to come out of the closet. The Procrustean bed is ancient history. If not now, when? What is standing the way? Who is the gatekeeper now?

> *"There is a vitality, a life force, a quickening*
> *that is translated through you into action,*
> *and because there is only one of you in all time,*
> *this expression is unique. If you block it, it will*
> *never exist through any other medium and be lost.*

The world will not have it.
It is not your business to determine how good
it is; nor how valuable it is; nor how it compares
with other expressions. It is your business to
keep it yours clearly and directly,
to keep the channel open.
You do not even have to believe in yourself or
your work. You have to keep open and aware
directly to the urges that motivate you.
Keep the channel open.

MARTHA GRAHAM

EXERCISING OUR POWER TO CHOOSE

Certain important realizations are associated with coming full cycle into the flourishing phase. Part of this is truly grasping the sacredness of the present moment and the embracing the opportunity to make the most of our precious human life. Transformative healing and growth in the face of adversity changes our relationship to what really matters. It brings to the forefront the question of what truly has meaning and purpose for us personally, right here and right now. Again, the calmer our mind and body is, the more we can see that we are surrounded by options and choices. Repetition for emphasis, it is in exercising our power to choose that we determine who we are and who we are becoming. This is something worth reminding ourselves of often.

Everything lies in the freedom of choice
that we possess as human beings.
Our liberation and our bondage.
There is no other species that has
the power to choose to evolve.

In light of this discovery, you have to ask yourself:
What am I doing with the gift of choice
that is my birthright as a human being?
ANDREW COHEN

The more we exercise our power to choose what has meaning and purpose for us, the more we will continue to thrive and flourish. In the face of fear and uncertainty, every time we connect with the good, the true, and the beautiful, we invest in our own spiritual endowment. Every time we see a need in the world and ask, "How can I help?" we nourish our own being while potentially contributing to the solution. This is where zest for life and passion come from. One of the few things that all spiritual traditions and most atheists agree on is that is it not what you get from life that matters but what you bring to it, for the benefit of others.

Existence will remain meaningless for you
Until you yourself penetrate into it with active love,
and in this way discover its meaning for yourself.
Everything is waiting to be hallowed by you.
Martin Buber

PORTALS TO THE SACRED

There is a wellspring within each of us, where our essential uniqueness meets our yearning to be and to become. Eight hundred years ago, the Sufi poet **Rumi** was saying, "There is a light-seed grain inside your soul. You fill it with yourself, or it dies."

These words reverberate to this day. When **Bob Dylan** sang, "He not busy being born is busy dying," he struck another unforgettable chord. It doesn't matter which portal we use to enter the sacred space of our own spiritual being—anything from music to nature to silence to the sea to prayer to belly dancing. It doesn't matter.

What matters is that we honor the gift of our own totally unique and unlikely and precious life by going there, hopefully often enough to keep our inner garden thriving—so that the weeds that threaten to choke the life out of us don't have their way with our sense of joy, so we can consciously choose which seeds we want to grow and nurture there, so we can clear the space, letting in all the light and rain and spiritual nourishment we need to thrive—knowing that in the end, the quality of our life depends on it.

> *If we fail to nourish our souls, they wither,*
> *and without soul, life ceases to have meaning.*
> *The creative process shrivels*
> *in the absence of continual dialogue with the soul.*
> *And creativity is what makes life worth living.*
>
> MARION WOODMAN

BLUEPRINT FOR FLOURISHING

Now that we have made it through the phases of transformative change, we find that we are consistently opening to a deeper level of conscious awareness. The everyday rewards of living this way tend to reinforce our more evolved way of seeing the world and our place in it. Our perspective has shifted and broadened. Given where we have been, we are relieved and grateful to be precisely where we are. Nonetheless, maintaining this newly established way of being always requires practice, self-observation, introspection, and occasional readjustment.

In summary, we enhance the chances that we will persevere in flourishing if we remain mindful of certain essentials and are using self-regulation skills when we need them. In *The Myths of Happiness*, by psychologist and author **Sonja Lyubomirsky**, professor of psychology at the University of California-Riverside, current research on basic happiness points to the importance of three areas:

- being emotionally connected to loved ones and having close and loving relationships with family and friends;
- having a strong sense of community and helping others in a meaningful way; and
- remaining committed to personal growth, using your gifts, and learning new things.

In addition, recent discoveries in neuroscience indicate that we can play a far more active role in increasing our emotional well-being than was previously understood.

NEUROSCIENCE AND POSITIVE EMOTIONS

Richard Davidson, Ph.D., professor of psychology and psychiatry at the University of Wisconsin–Madison, has been leading cutting-edge research in this area for decades at the Laboratory for Affective Neuroscience, Waisman Laboratory for Brain Imaging and Behavior, and the Center for Investigating Healthy Minds. He and his colleagues are currently using positron emission tomography (PET) and functional magnetic resonance imaging (fMRI) to study, among other things, the short-term and long-term impact of meditation practice on the brain.

Davidson's research, particularly on the prefrontal cortex, is demonstrating a positive impact on our capacity for experiencing and sustaining all positive emotions, including happiness, empathy, peacefulness, loving kindness, and compassion. The left prefrontal cortex is also the area of the brain that appears to play an important role in creativity.

Again, meditation practice does make a difference. Whether we regard it as spiritual practice or relaxation training is not the point. In its most direct, experiential form, spiritual practice can simply mean living more mindfully with greater attention to the present on a moment-to-moment basis with nonjudgmental awareness.

It can also include making the decision to set aside even 15 minutes of quiet time on a regular basis, preferably daily, to practice calming the body and quieting the mind, for the physical and emotional benefits of deep relaxation as well as for the purpose of enhancing insight, wisdom, creativity, and spiritual growth.

COGNITIVE RESTRUCTURING IN A NUTSHELL

As discussed earlier, thanks to breathing techniques and increased body awareness, we can learn to catch ourselves early and intervene on our own behalf, releasing tension and creating the inner space necessary to make the shift from a negative automatic thought to more realistic appraisal of the situation. This is cognitive restructuring in its most basic form:

1. noticing what emotion you're feeling;
2. noticing the thought that has led to this emotion;
3. challenging the validity of that thought; and then
4. choosing a more accurate view of what is actually happening.

Why is this so important? Because we feel the way we think. When we change the way we think, we change the way we feel. And when we change our thought, we change our physiology as well as our emotional state. This is the pivotal piece. Just as we release anxiety with a few deep cleansing breaths, the possibility of cognitive reframing becomes a more feasible option. Until we lower our anxiety level through deep breathing, conscious choice remains less available or simply unavailable to us.

The next goal is to shed light on our own habitual way of thinking so that we can readily see where it is distorted, illogical, or exaggerated. Even the most highly functioning individuals have some blind spots, some areas where the reality of a situation is somehow obscured by their hidden biases and flawed perceptions. According to **David D. Burns, MD**, who introduced *Cognitive Behavioral Therapy* in the 1980s, the most common *cognitive distortions* are—

1. all-or-nothing thinking: looking at things in absolute, black-or-white categories
2. over-generalizing: viewing a single negative event as a never-ending pattern of defeat
3. mental filtering: dwelling on the negatives and ignoring the positives
4. discounting the positives: insisting that your accomplishments or positive qualities don't count
5. jumping to conclusions: concluding things are bad without any definite evidence:
6. mind-reading: assuming someone is reacting negatively toward you
7. fortune-telling: predicting that things will turn out badly
8. magnifying or minimizing: blowing things way out of proportion or shrinking their importance
9. emotional reasoning: considering your emotional feeling to be evidence of the truth. ("I'm feeling overwhelmed, so I must be a helpless person.")
10. "should" statements: criticizing yourself or others with shoulds and shouldn'ts, musts, oughts, and have-tos.
11. labeling: name calling (toward self). Instead of saying, "I made a mistake," you tell yourself "I can't believe I am such an idiot."
12. personalizing and self-blaming: assuming responsibility for a negative event (how someone else behaves, for example) that was beyond your control
13. what if… what if…[our worst imaginings of what might happen]
14. perfectionism: it must be perfect or it isn't okay, worthwhile, enough,

Do you see yourself in any of those? Several of them? All of them? Instead of being taken in, oppressed, depressed, or even tyrannized a by negative thought that is probably not even accurate to begin with, we can develop the ability to question any thought that seems to be triggering an intense emotional reaction in us. Often, just asking the question is evidence that we are dealing with a cognitive distortion.

To make the shift from emotionally charged subjective thinking (where we are held captive within the grips of the negative emotion, also known as an emotional hijack) to more rational, objective thinking (where we can step back and hold the emotion from a distance), it helps to get in the habit of asking these questions. It's about reestablishing self-command, which is always a good idea.

Questions for reframing:
- Is this really true, or am I jumping to conclusions?
- Is this thought really helping me right now, or am I catastrophizing?
- Is this helping me to move forward, or is it keeping me stuck?
- Is it to my advantage to think this way, or is there another way to look at the situation?
- Is it really as bad as it seems? If it is, does it pay to give it so much attention?

Once we've replaced an inaccurate habitual thought with a more rational and constructive one, it can be helpful to choose an affirmation as a way of establishing an encouraging and calm frame of mind. Affirmations are positive statements, designed to counter negative thinking. They are free and easy and universally helpful. Repeating them can bring about important changes in how we think and feel. Ideally, we will create our very own affirmations that more specifically reflect our best vision. Here are some generic examples of **affirmations** that many people find supportive:
- I deeply accept and love myself, exactly as I am.
- I am able to feel grateful for my many blessings.
- I am more and more able to relax my body and calm my mind.

- I can handle it. This too shall pass.
- I can let go of negativity and hold on to what really matters.
- I am dearly loved and capable of great loving.

Releasing negative emotions as they arise is essential for maintaining enough enthusiasm and balance to keep us on the journey, following the path of living in accordance with our truest truth. Every life will have more than its share of adversity, as we all well know. However, adversity is not the problem. Our habitual way of reacting to adversity is the problem. The more we work constructively and diligently with this fact, the freer, more liberated, and happier we become. The more awareness we have regarding our ingrained patterns, the more effective we will be at releasing ourselves from them.

EVERYDAY ADVERSITY AND THE SPIRITUAL WARRIOR

Making it through these steps is about triumphing over major adversity, evolving as a person, becoming wiser, freer, more resilient, compassionate, loving, and more consciously aware—in short, experiencing a heightened sense of well-being. But what about the future difficulties that we will all continue to encounter throughout our lives? Obviously hardship cannot be prevented from occurring in the form of troubling external challenges and painful emotional states that come to us in waves, unwelcome and unbidden. But there they are.

We know there is no protection from unpreventable forms of inner and outer adversity coming our way. But we also now know that there is one thing we can always do. We can live a more mindful and evolved life by meeting these ongoing challenges with the insights, tools, confidence, awareness and resilience of a spiritual warrior who has learned how to skillfully handle whatever happens next.

UNIVERSAL PHENOMENON

Even when our life is humming along with just familiar everyday stuff going on, we can be hit with a wave of fear or sadness or outrage that sends us reeling. This is a universal phenomenon. To expect uninterrupted happiness from any life, no matter how blessed, is simply unrealistic. What makes the difference is how we handle it when it comes.

Rather than compounding the pain by being hard on ourselves for feeling miserable (fearful, insecure, resentful, envious, angry, sorrowful, rejected, unloved, like a failure, whatever) the goal is to notice what is happening as soon as possible. Then go back to the stages and steps outlined in the book, locate where we are in the sequence, and use whatever tools, practices, insights, or exercises are needed to carry us onward and forward.

Now and then, what we need most is a quick fix, either to pull us out of a funk in a hurry or to get us over a hump with a negative state that keeps showing up at the wrong time despite our best efforts to get past it. This exercise is a great one to have in **our spiritual tool bag**:

EXERCISE: QUICK FIX FOR RELEASING NEGATIVE EMOTION

* What emotion are you feeling right now? Name it; acknowledge it.
* Where [in your body] do you feel this feeling?
* In theory, can you let it go? Could someone else let it go?
* Will you let go of it? Are you planning to, eventually?
* When will you let go of it? Now? Not now?
* Not now? Then ask yourself: would you rather continue feeling this way? Or would you rather be free?

IN CONCLUSION: THE ULTIMATE CHALLENGE

This book is about our relationship to change. It is an impassioned invitation to become actively engaged in all the areas of our life that are truly within our ability to control. But what about the many aspects that are simply beyond our control? Obviously they are endless—not just the monumental issues beyond our realm of influence, but the everyday worries, disappointments, resentments, uncertainties, frustrations, impasses. When it's possible to respond constructively, that is one thing. We do what we can. Fine.

But what about the nagging concerns and regrets, the all too familiar thoughts that are *not* a call to action at all, just a painful rehash of old material? Cumulatively, this kind of unwitting rumination can take our life hostage, making us a prisoner of our thoughts. It can dampen our optimism and drain our energy. It can effectively block us from savoring our life, let alone fulfilling our destiny. "Even the lion must defend himself from the gnats," as the saying goes.

The good news is that this problem is workable, for many reasons. In fact, this very negativity, the chronic emotional suffering that threatens to vaporize our sense of peace and joy, can be the catalyst to seriously making meditation practice part of our everyday life. This is probably one of the most important choices we could make—and not just from the standpoint of emotional freedom, personal development, and spiritual growth.

As discussed earlier, the physical benefits of meditation have been well-documented across a broad spectrum that includes cardiovascular, neuroendocrine, neuromuscular, immunological, etc. We now have more than 40 years of hard science confirming meditation's positive impact on our physiology.

Harvard cardiologist **Herbert Benson, MD**, author of *The Relaxation Response*, first introduced meditation to western medicine in the 1970s. Although Benson conducted extensive research with Buddhist monks adept at meditating, he presented his findings in a strictly clinical context to gain acceptance within the scientifically oriented medical community. Benson kept the language culture-free, describing meditation as a practical stress-reduction technique capable of eliciting the relaxation response, which of course it is.

The technique involved simply taking a short break in a quiet safe place, temporarily letting go of distractions and concerns, opening to the present moment, and focusing one's attention on the flow of the breath. Today meditation is regarded in integrative medicine as an effective self-care tool, an evidence-based intervention recommended by physicians worldwide.

An easily acquired skill set, meditation has been clinically proven to significantly improve psychological and emotional well-being. Benson's colleague, molecular biologist and Zen practitioner **Jon Kabat-Zinn, Ph.D.**, continued his research with patients, developing and founding mindfulness-based stress-reduction programs in 1979. These life-changing eight-week seminars are being conducted worldwide to this day.

Zinn's first book, *Full Catastrophe Living: Using the Wisdom of your Body and Mind to face Stress, Pain, and Illness*, was published in 1991, changing public policy on patient education and self-care forever. During the last 40 years, thanks to the pioneering work of Benson, Zinn, Davidson, and others, the multi-level benefits of meditation have been recognized and embraced by hospitals, medical schools worldwide, and by the general public in ever increasing numbers.

WITNESS CONSCIOUSNESS IN MEDITATION AND IN LIFE

Aside from improving our physical well-being and enhancing our capacity to experience positive emotional states, both short term and long term—literally changing neural circuitry in our brains for the better—one of the most important benefits of having a regular meditation practice is the gradual development of what is sometimes referred to as *witness consciousness*.

It's about being fully present and, at the same time, calmly bearing witness to whatever we are experiencing. Just as mindfulness is central to increasing awareness, witness consciousness can be thought of as a transcendent form of mindfulness. Both can be naturally cultivated through the practice of meditation.

During meditation, the witness is the aspect of our mind that is able to observe thoughts and images as they come and go, without getting caught up in them. Witnessing begins as focused awareness in the body, through noticing the rhythm of our breathing and our bodily sensations without critiquing anything, but rather just observing the continuous flow of feelings, thoughts, and sensations with a deeper and deeper realization that they are all impermanent anyway. No thought has solidity, no feeling is final.

Realizing this, the body begins to relax, and tension softens, which lays the foundation for clarity, discernment, and wisdom to spontaneously come forth. Witness consciousness is our capacity for maintaining what Indian philosopher **Jiddu Krishnamurti** called *"choiceless awareness,"* the ability to remain grounded and centered, allowing positive and negative thoughts to flow through us without reacting to them.

Witness consciousness can serve as our loyal companion and spiritual bodyguard as we naturally increase our ability to maintain a sense of abiding calm, physically and emotionally. Again, thanks to neuroplasticity, every time we repeat this practice, it gets a little easier. We are building resilience and stress-hardiness on deeper and deeper levels.

Through direct experience in meditation, we come to know firsthand that we each have our own inner sanctuary. We come to recognize that there is a peaceful, silent dimension within us that has remained intact and unscathed, regardless of anything and everything that has ever happened to us or ever will.

Each time we practice letting go of a thought and bringing our attention back to the flow of the breath, we liberate ourselves a little more from deeply ingrained negative thought patterns. The more we focus our attention on our breath in this very moment, the more skillful we become at witnessing how our mind works and then exercising our power to consciously choose this lighter, freer, more enlightened way of being, again and again. Getting better at letting go is about becoming freer and freer from the inside out.

From this awareness and understanding comes a certain confidence that we can extricate ourselves from whatever it is that oppresses us: fear, sorrow, anger, resentment, regret, despair, etc. This faith in ourselves, along with a deepening understanding of impermanence, enables us to cultivate a sense of equanimity in the face of uncertainty, change, loss, etc.

This is more than a life skill. It is a spiritual strength that enables us to flourish because now we can endure life's vicissitudes without contracting in fear, withdrawing, lashing out or shutting down. Instead, we can remain totally present and be with what is happening long enough to ride each wave as we continue to embrace life wholeheartedly.

Going forward, our most constructive action comes from being grounded in relaxed awareness. When we truly inhabit our body, as opposed to being stuck in our head with its convincing story, we have fuller access to clarity and wisdom. Our perceptions are informed by our heart and our gut as well as our best cognitive abilities.

This facilitates discernment and the possibility of right action. Choiceless awareness or witness consciousness allows us to clearly see the next right thing to do in any given situation. No constriction, no grasping, no judging, no pushing away. Just observing the energy flowing in and through us and out of us again.

Softening into the present moment, we are trusting the process with no past and no future, just this inhale, just this exhale. Day by day, breath by breath, conscious choice is more and more available. There is peace and joy and great freedom in this practice. At first, we may make an effort to meditate just to minimize pain. Then we do it to experience peace.

Then we practice out of sheer self-loyalty, so we can actualize our potential and live our dream.

But ultimately, we do this work for the benefit of others because the more joy and freedom and compassion we experience toward ourselves, the more our presence and our actions will be of benefit to loved ones, friends, strangers, the world. In the end, it's about coming home to ourselves. It's about opening to this precious gift of life, with all its blessings and adversities, dialing down the noise, and tuning into what really matters today, here and now, and always being ready to realign our life in accordance with what is true for us, even in the tiniest of increments.

It's about investigating our life from time to time and sorting it all out: *discerning* between what we want versus what we are truly *yearning* for. And then bringing this understanding and self-awareness to consciousness more and more. It's about releasing ourselves from the inevitable restrictions of past conditioning, overcoming our internal resistance, managing our obstacles, and giving ourselves permission to honor what the "still small voice inside" has to say to us by deeply listening to it. And then focusing on giving birth to a life, labor pains and all, our one sacred life, based on what has meaning and purpose for us.

It's about inviting an image to form in our mind of how and where we'd love to be — visualizing already being there with all of our five senses until it becomes more and more real to us. And then gradually, imperceptibly, moment by moment, against all odds, in the light and in the dark, bringing it forth into the world: becoming the hero of our own story. And then we will live well, and we will die well. And that is what flourishing is about.

The Holy Longing
I praise what is truly alive ...
And so long as you haven't experienced this:

To die and so to grow
You are only a troubled guest on the dark earth
GOETHE

SUMMARY POINTS: CHAPTER 7:
EVOLVING—FLOURISHING

"I wish no one had to suffer, but in my case
it was an important catalyst to my growth;
I am more grateful, humble, connected, loving, and
really fearless, etc. than I ever thought possible."
EXCERPT FROM CASE STUDY

Cognition: I am thriving. Pain can be a gateway to liberation. I am in the flow. This is how it feels to flourish, to emerge.

Premise: Pain cannot be eliminated, but it can provide motivation for transforming my life and increasing conscious awareness.

NAT → RRR: I can handle whatever happens; I can use it as a springboard. I can liberate myself and others. (NATs are recognized and replaced with RRRs.)

Emotions: joy, equanimity, confidence, optimism, exuberant sense of abiding calm, choiceless awareness, peace, gratitude, moment-to-moment awareness and joyful exertion; mindfulness, emotional freedom

Physical: with increasing ease, maintaining optimum wellness, balanced energy, stress hardiness, resilience; healthy lifestyle is self-motivating.

Behavioral: creative, constructive, more conscious individually; more connected, cooperative, collaborative in a larger context; practicing meditation

Spiritual: in this world but not of this world; the Procrustean bed

Realization: a new sense of meaning and purpose. I can practice meditation. I can exercise freedom of choice. This is "my one wild and precious life."

Catalysts and Impediments:

Potential Pitfall: "Don't go back to sleep." RUMI

Blueprint for Flourishing: personal growth, connection with loved ones, sense of community, making a contribution to the well-being of others; spiritual practice, including meditation, introspection, reflection; releasing negative emotions to maintain enthusiasm and balance; visualization of best self, living in accordance with one's truth.

CHAPTER 8

Transformational Change—A Global Perspective

*In the history of the collective
as in the history of the individual,
everything depends on
the development of consciousness.*

CARL JUNG

GLOBAL ADVERSITY, THRESHOLD, AND CRITICAL MASS

Tying the phenomenology of change in a human life span into the concept of transformation in the culture, we see many of the same dynamics. At present, there is growing awareness worldwide of the magnitude of our environmental, economic, political, health, and social problems as well as the nagging sense that, despite the rhetoric of our political analysts, corporate leaders, and social commentators, the situation is only getting worse. At the same time, there is a huge conspiracy of denial, partly due to conflicts of interest (corporate, economic, political), a certain public apathy, and the consensus trance of contemporary life, most of which is fueled by our institutionalized addiction to greed and maintained by a myopic ignorance of the consequences.

The current crises represent a critical time of acute adversity where our previous approaches, our worn-out tools and strategies have failed to rectify the problems, despite our best efforts within the existing system of premises and beliefs. Where is this going? Hopefully, with increasing readiness within individuals and collectively within cultures, it is headed toward a tipping point. This dynamic of reaching a threshold or critical mass is just as observable in the current transformation in global consciousness as it is in a single individual's life span. Backing up as far as the earliest eras in cosmic evolution, we have seen how the Earth has moved through an ongoing sequence of crises that threatened its very existence, from the Cambrian extinction phase 570 million years ago when probably 85 percent of all species were destroyed to a whole series of subsequent life-threatening devolutions, through which shifts occurred and solutions emerged.

The earth's ability to endure has so effectively been demonstrated that theoretical physicists, such as **Peter Russell**, author of *Waking Up in Time*, have come to regard the universe as a living, unfolding entity with the consciousness to save itself. Science has definitively observed that the transformative pattern of evolution involves self-regulation through shifts and consequent reorganizations, progressing toward more complex levels of evolution.

In *Microcosmos: Four Billion Years of Microbial Evolution*, microbiologists **Lynn Margulis and Dorian Sagan** have observed that a form of consciousness or intelligence involving self-regulation is just as evident in certain highly conserved microbes as it is in the cosmos. They have been maintaining life by identifying danger—a new antibiotic formulated to kill it, for example—and responding to that antibiotic in a life preserving manner: by changing, literally unbraiding themselves and rebraiding in a different configuration to render the antibiotic harmless to them. Microbes have been moving toward a source of energy (food and light) for literally billions of years now.

What's amazing to consider is that this very same pattern of life sustained, life threatened, chaos, emergence, and evolution can be playing itself out within our own life span. The good news is that, to the extent that we can regard our difficulties as important opportunities, as grist for our personal transformation, we can relate to even our most painful crises as our most valuable growth experiences.

UNRAVELING OUTMODED PARADIGMS

Just as we have seen the in the model for human transformation, a phase of further deterioration eventually leads to a breaking point, a bottoming out, in which old patterns and defenses begin to crumble and openness to change first becomes possible. In global economics, for example, this has become increasingly evident. Economic policies that were logical and justifiable a hundred years ago are now understood as unsustainable, due to the inescapable realities we are now confronting: global warming, the energy crisis, the depletion of nonrenewable resources and their destructive impact on the environment and on our quality of life.

Although the mainstream response to these crises continues to be partially one of denial, information exchange is rapidly occurring, pressure is mounting, and growing awareness is now unstoppable. We, as a global culture are gradually waking up to the enormity of the problem.

TURNING POINTS: SHIFTING PERSPECTIVES

What are some of the possibilities that may be lying ahead? In the short term, we are looking at more obliviousness and denial in the face of mounting evidence, increasing deterioration, movement toward critical mass, and further approaches to the threshold for significant change. Visionary leaders from Einstein and Gandhi to Vaclav Havel and Martin Luther King affirmed for years that this is the time for transcendence to a higher consciousness.

Yet out of the rubble and crumbling of the post-modern age, we are still in the process of transitioning toward a major shift in fundamental values,

toward the birth of new meaning. Enlightened spiritual leaders from the
Dalai Lama to contemporary philosophers like Ken Wilber and pragmatic
luminaries like economist-political activist-social prophet Jeremy Rifkin
share this vision for a new world order, calling for transcendence to our
shared humanity and spiritual interconnectedness. They and others too
numerous to mention see it as the only realistic alternative to extinction.

It's going to take a profound spiritual renewal in which the miracle of
life itself and the vital importance of a global perspective is honored by
all people.

Self-transcendence is as crucial to the process of human evolution as it
is to global consciousness. This is the shift in perspective that will carry us
through the turning point, cultivating the spiritual dimension and realizing transcendence, individually and collectively, within the global community in which our future survival is held.

We do have the option to make it.
Either you're going to go along with your mind and the truth,
or you're going to yield
to fear and custom and conditioned reflexes.
With our minds alone we can discover those principles we need
to employ to convert all humanity to success
in a new, harmonious relationship with the universe.

R. BUCKMINSTER FULLER

My profound hope is that reading this book will be a catalyst in some
way to your own inherent capacity for transformative growth. May you
approach life's challenges with enough awareness, insight, resilience, and
skill to courageously meet whatever inevitable crisis lies ahead. And may
you effectively transform it into the next leap forward in your own personal evolution.

INDEX

BIBLIOGRAPHY

Abram, D. (1997). Spell of the Sensuous. New York: Random House.

Abram, J. (1996). The Language of Winnecott. London: H. Karmac Books, Ltd.

Arrien, A. (1993). The Fourfold Way. New York: Harper Collins.

Austin, J. H. (1998). Zen and the Brain. Cambridge: MIT Press.

Baars, B. (1997). In the Theater of Consciousness. New York: Oxford University Press.

Beck, C.J. (1993). Nothing Special: Living Zen. New York: Harper Collins.

Benson, H. et al. (1997). Spirituality & Healing in Medicine-IV. Harvard Medical School Mind/Body Medical Institute.

Benson, H. et al. (1999). Clinical Training in Mind/Body Medicine: Provider's Manual. Harvard University Printing and Publishing

Benson, H., Klipper, M. (1992) The Relaxation Response. Wing Books

Benson, H. (2015) Mind Body Effect: How to Counteract the Harmful Effects of Stress. New York: Simon & Schuster

Berry, T. (1988). The Dream of the Earth. San Francisco: Sierra Club Books.

Bohm, David. (1980). Wholeness and the Implicate Order. London: Routeledge.

Bolen, J. S. (1996). Close to the Bone. New York: Scribner.

Boreysenko, J. (1993). Fire in the Soul. New York: Warner.

Braud, W. & Anderson, R. (1998) Transpersonal Research Methods for the Social Sciences. London: Sage

Campbell, J. (1964). Occidental Mythology: The Masks of God. New York: Penguin.

Capra, F. (1982). TheTurning Point. New York: Simon and Schuster.

Capra, F. (1996). The Web of Life. New York: Harper Collins.

Carnes, R. D. & Craig, S. (1998). Sacred Circles. New York: Harper Collins.

Caudhill, M. A. (1995). Managing Pain Before it Manages You. New York: Guilford Press.

Chodron, P. (1991). The Wisdom of No Escape. Boston: Shambala.

Csikszentmihalyi, M. (1991). Flow. New York: Harper Collins.
_____(1993). The Evolving Self. New York: Harper Collins.
Dalai Lama, et.al. (1991). MindScience: An East-West Dialogue. Boston: Wisdom Publications.
Davidson,RJ, Begley,S. (2012) The Emotional Life of Your Brain. New York: Hudson Street Press
Eccles, J., MD. (1994). How the Self Controls the Brain. Heidleberg: Springer-Verlag
Eisler, R. (1987). The Chalice and the Blade. New York: Harper Collins.
Eisler, R. & Loye, D. (1990). The Partnership Way. New York: Harper Collins.
Eldridge, N. 1998). Life in the Balance. Princeton University Press.
Elgin, D. (1997). Global Consciousness Change. San Anselmo, CA: Millenium.
Epstein, M. (1998). Going to Pieces Without Falling Apart. New York: Bantam.
Farthing. G.W. (1992). The Psychology of Consciousness. Englewood Cliffs, NJ: Prentice-Hall
Ferrini, P. (1996). The Silence of the Heart. Deerfield, MA: Heartways Press.
Frankl, V. (1959). Man's Search for Meaning. New York: Simon & Schuster.
Fredrickson, B. (2009). Positivity:Top-Notch Research Reveals 3 to 1 Ratio That Will Change Your Life. New York: Harmony (2013). Love 2.0: How Our Supreme Emotion Affects Everything We Feel, Think, Do, and Become. New York: Avery
Gimbutas, M. (1989). The Language of the Goddess. London: Thames & Hudson, Ltd.
Goenka, S. N. (1987). The Discourse Summaries. Maharashtra, India: Vipashyana Vinyas
Goswami, A. (1999). Quantum Creativity. New Jersey: Hampton Press.
Halifax, J. (1993). The Fruitful Darkness. New York: Harper Collins.
Harmon, W. (1998). Global Mind Change. San Fraancisco: Berrett-Keohler.
Havel, V. (1994). A time for trandscendence. Philadelphia: lecture.
Henderson, H. (1991). Paradigms in Progress. Indianapolis: Knowledge Systems.
_____ (1996). Building a Win-Win World. SanFrancisco: Berrett-Keohler.
Hubbard, B.M. (1998). Conscious Evolution. Novato, CA: New World Library.
Hunt, H.T. (1995). On the Nature of Consciousness: Cognitive, Phenomenological, and Transpersonal Perspectives. NewHaven: Yale University Press
Jaidar, G. (1995). The Soul. New York: Paragon House
Jung, C.G.   (1968) Man and His Symbols. New York: Dell Publishing
              (1989) Memories, Dreams, Reflections Vintage (reissue)

(1993) The Basic Writings of C. G. Jung. Modern Library

(2006) The Undiscovered Self. Berkley (reissue)

Kabat-Zinn, J. (1990). Full Catastrophe Living. New York: Doubleday

_____(1994). Wherever You Go There You Are. New York: Hyperion.

1.1.1.1 (2005). Coming to Our Senses: Healing Ourselves and the World Through Mindfulness.

Koenig, H. MD (1999). The Healing Power of Faith. New York: Simon & Schuster.

Kornfield, J. (1993). A Path with Heart. New York: Bantam.

Le Shan, L. (1989). Cancer as a Turning Point. New York: E. P. Dutton

Levine, P. (1997). Walking the Tiger: Healing Trauma. Berkeley: North Atlantic Books.

Lyubomirsky, S. (2008) The How of Happiness. New York: Penguin Press (2013) The Myth of Happiness. New York: Penguin Press

Margoles, L., Sagan, D., Thomas, L. (1997). Microcosmos. University of California Press.

McCormick, E. (1997). Living on the Edge. Rockport, MA: Element Books.

Mitchell, S. Trans. (1988). Tao Te Ching. New York: Harper and Row.

Nhat Hanh, T. (1991). Peace is Every Step:The Path of Mindfulness in Everyday life. New York: Putnam

_____(1999). The Heart of the Buddha's Teaching. Berkeley: Parallax Press.

O'Donohue, J. (1997). Anam Cara. New York: Harper Collins.

Omai, K. (1999). The Borderless World: Power and Strategy in the Interlinked Economy. New York:Harpers.

Pearce, J. (1993). Evolution's End: Claiming the Potential of Our Intelligence. San Francisco: Harper.

Peck, M. S. (1987). The Different Drum. New York: Simon and Schuster.

Pennebaker, J. (1990). Opening Up: The Healing Power of Expressing Emotions. New York: Guilford Press

Pert, C. (1997). Molecules of Emotion. New York: Touchstone.

Phillips, A. (1988). Winnecott. Cambridge: Harvard University Press.

Rechtshafen, S. (1996). Timeshifting. New York: Doubleday.

Reps, P. (1957). Zen Flesh, Zen Bones. Tokyo: Charles Tuttle Company

Rinposhe, S. (1993). The Tibetan Book of Living and Dying. New York: Harper Collins.

Rogers, E. M. (1995). Diffusion of Innovations. New York: Simon and Schuster

Rosen, D, MD (1993). Transforming Depression: Healing the Soul through Creativity. New York: Putnam

Roszak, T. (1993). Voice of the Earth. Portland, OR: Touchstone Press.

Rossman, MD, M.L., (2000) Guided Imagery for Self-Healing. HJ Kramer/New World Library

Rothberg, D. & Kelly, S., Ed. (1998). Ken Wilber in Dialogue. Wheaton, IL: Quest Books.

Russell, P. (1992). The White Hole in Time. London: The Aquarian Press.

_____ (1998). Waking Up in Time, London: Origin Press

Searle, J.R. (1997). The Mystery of Consciousness. New York: NY Review of Books.

Seligman, M.E.P. (2011) Flourish. New York: Simon and Schuster

Schoenowolf, G. (1990). Turning Points in Analytic Therapy. London: Jason Aronson.

Sheldrake, R. (1991). The Rebirth of Nature. Rochester, VT: Park Street Press.

_____ (1981). A New Science of Life. Los Angeles: P. Tarcher

_____ (1995). The Presence of the Past. London: Inner Traditions, Ltd.

Sivaraska, S. (1992). Seeds of Peace: a Buddhist vision for Renewing society. Bangkok: Ruen Kaew Press.

Smith, H. (1994). The Illustrated World's Religions. New York: Harper Collins.

Smullyan, R. (1977). The Tao is Silent. New York: Harper Collins.

Sturgeon, N. (1997). Ecofeminist Natures. New York: Routledge.

Suzuki, S. (1975). Zen Mind, Beginner's Mind. New York: Walker/Weatherhill.

Swimme, B. & Berry, T. (1992). The Universe Story. New York: Harper Collins.

Tart, C. (1986). Waking Up. Shambala: Boston

Tart, C. Ed. (1997) Body Mind Spirit. Charlottesville: Hampton Roads.

Tarrant, J. (1998). The Light Inside the Dark. New York: Harper

Thondup, T. (1996). The Healing Power of Mind. Boston: Shambala.

Thurman, R. (1998). Inner Revolution. New York: Riverhead Books.

_____ (1997). Essential Tibetan Buddhism. New Jersey: Castle Books.

Trungpa, C. (1973). Cutting Through Spiritual Materialism. Boston: Shambala

_____ (1995). The Path is the Goal. Boston: Shambala

U Pandita, S. (1991). In This Very Life. Kandy, Sri Lanka: Buddhist Publication Society.

Valle, R. Ed., (1998). Phenomenological Inquiry in Psychology: Existential and Transpersonal Perspectives. Yale University Press.

Velmans, M.,Ed. (1997). The Science of Consciousness. London: Routledge.

Walker, A. (1997). Anything We Love Can Be Saved. New York: Random House.

Walsh, R. MD & Vaughan,F., Ed. (1993). Paths Beyond Ego: The Transpersonal Vision. New York: Putnam

Walsh, R. MD (1999). Essential Spirituality. New York: John Wiley & Sons.

Watts, A. (1983). The Way of Liberation. New York: Weatherhill.

Weil, A. (1995). Spontaneous Healing. New York: Ballantine.

_____ (1997). Roots of Healing, Carlsbad, CA: New Dimensions.

Wenk, H.E. (1997). The effect of concentrative attention on habitual cognition. Unpublished Dissertation, Yale University.

Wetzel, M.S.; Eisenberg, D.M.; & Kaptchuk, T.J. (1998) Courses involving complementary and alternative medicine at US medical schools. Journal of the American Medical Association, 280, 784-787.

Whitmyer, C. Ed. (1994). Mindfulness and Meaningful Work. Berkeley, CA: Parallax Press.

Whyte, D. (1996). The Heart Aroused. New York: Doubleday.

Wilber, K. (1990). The Atman Project. Wheaton, IL: Quest Books.

_____ (1996). A Brief History of Everything. Boston: Shambala.

_____ (1998). The Essential Ken Wilber. Boston: Shambala.

_____ (1998). The Marriage of Sense and Soul. New York: Random House.

Wilber, K., Engler, J. & Brown, D. (1986). Transformations of Consciousness. Boston: Shambala

Woolf, V. (1938). Three Guineas. New York: Harcourt Brace.

Young-Eisenrath, P. (1996). The Resilient Spirit. Reading, MA: Addison Wesley.

Made in the USA
Columbia, SC
09 December 2020

27073380R00115